Yoga of Resilience

Yoga of Resilience

*Embodying a Practice
to Thrive Through Hardship*

KELLY B. GOLDEN

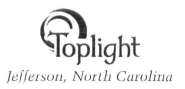

Jefferson, North Carolina

All illustrations are by Scott Howard.

LIBRARY OF CONGRESS CATALOGUING-IN-PUBLICATION DATA

Names: Golden, Kelly B., 1977– author.
Title: Yoga of resilience : embodying a practice to thrive through hardship /
Kelly B. Golden.
Description: Jefferson, North Carolina : Toplight, 2023 | Includes bibliographical
references and index.
Identifiers: LCCN 2022059063 | ISBN 9781476687223 (paperback : acid free paper) ∞
ISBN 9781476648675 (ebook)
Subjects: LCSH: Yoga. | Resilience (Personality trait) | Self-actualization (Psychology)
Classification: LCC B132.Y6 .G5835 2023 | DDC 181/.45—dc23/eng/20230103
LC record available at https://lccn.loc.gov/2022059063

BRITISH LIBRARY CATALOGUING DATA ARE AVAILABLE

ISBN (print) 978-1-4766-8722-3
ISBN (ebook) 978-1-4766-4867-5

Front cover photograph by J.R. Berry;
background Shutterstock

Printed in the United States of America

Toplight is an imprint of McFarland & Company, Inc., Publishers

Box 611, Jefferson, North Carolina 28640
www.toplightbooks.com

For Dharma and Pippa,
the most inspiring and resilient people I know,
and to Bob and Mitzi for providing
the tools and support.

Contents

Preface

A perfect example of the divine play of the universe (*lila*) was offered to me three-quarters of the way through the completion of this book. As I was wrapping up the last chapter, I was faced with a monumental test of my own resilience. My father was diagnosed with end-stage lung cancer and sent home to receive hospice care through the end of his days. The journey was intense albeit quick. He was more alive than ever the first month and a half, then he began rapidly and steadily declining. He took his last breath on the morning of my 44th birthday, a week shy of four months post diagnosis. I was fortunate. I was able to step away from my business, leaving it in the highly capable hands of my long-time program coordinator. I was able to take a six-month sabbatical from teaching in order to give the necessary time to my family. I lived only about an hour away, so I was able to visit often, which transitioned to daily visits in the end. Our family was able to rally around him and help him to feel, in his own words, "washed in love."

During the time we had, we were all able to set aside our small irritations and fully immerse ourselves in the experience of supporting my father's transition, doing whatever we needed to assist in his comfort and care. My mother, daughters, godmother, and I moved into a place of presence together, holding him and each other in a loving space of sorrow right up to the end. We were blessed beyond measure to participate in one of the most important transitions of a life: its end.

As expected, the grief that followed was a heavy sadness mixed paradoxically with joyful remembering, full of laughter and many tears. My sorrow emerged from love rather than loss, as I believe that my father will continue on through my attending to his memory, his stories, his life well lived. Now, I find myself in the interesting position of putting the suggestions I have made in this book to the test, immediately and intensely.

I sit here now, having just finished eating a sandwich of tomatoes my father planted in his garden in the spring. My dining room table is adorned with the colorful zinnias that have grown from seeds he collected last year

1

then scattered haphazardly across the yard in the spring, a yard that is now alive and bursting with blooms. Most days, I think of him with almost every breath. Memories from long ago rise like cream in coffee to the top of my awareness. His life was full; he was an inspiration and a character to many. He knew love, maybe not perfectly but openly, gushingly, and proudly. He knew how to have fun, as story after story at his memorial showed, and he knew struggle, pain, disease, loss, fear, challenge. He had the full gamut. He was not spared his lot in life; he was blessed with it. He was far from perfect but spot on in his love.

This experience brought me fully and honestly into the work of resilience, and I won't lie and say I went willingly. Truth be told, I went kicking and screaming into the discomfort, applying all my old strategies of denial until I could no longer hide from the pain and heartache of the situation. The point of surrender was pivotal, and I allowed myself to enter the liminality of ending. I could be nowhere other than exactly where I was. I could not force my head above the waves of sadness, frustration, and fear, yet I did find myself ricocheting out of the swirl periodically for very brief moments. Overall, my inner rhythm slowed down, as sadness requires, and my tolerance receded. I was often overcome with frustration and pain that I had a difficult time understanding myself, much less expressing to others. The beauty that emerged alongside the pain was undeniable, but life became (and to some degree still is) weighty and full of challenge.

A few weeks after the memorial service for my father, I explained to a friend that it felt as if I had been carrying a very heavy backpack full of stones every day since the diagnosis, but until my dad passed, I was completely unaware of it. I was overloaded, laboring to put one foot in front of the other, and I didn't fully realize it. Sure, I was cognizant of my story, and I was aware of the intensity of my day-to-day life, but I was in it completely, unable to gain perspective on the situation in which I was immersed. Most aspects of my life began to feel flat and hard. The practices and processes that I encourage you to explore in this book weren't available to me during this time. My meditation became routine; my āsana practice became an escape. My personal relationships suffered. I withdrew into the tiny bubble of my family, and together, we became fully absorbed in the lamentation. I was in it, and it wasn't okay. It was sad and scary, hard and heavy. And *not* wrong. Nor was it something to attempt to get out of. It was simply and exactly where I was. Only now am I beginning to access the buoyancy of resilience. Only now, after the painful process of bearing witness to the passing of one of the most important people in my life, can I begin to respond to it.

2

Preface

You see, resilience is a way to rebound from struggle, not to escape from it. When you are in the struggle, you are struggling, and you aren't necessarily resilient. It's in the aftermath of struggle that resilience emerges. So, please, as you begin this book, know that these pages do not suggest a way out of your difficulties and struggles, but rather they offer a path to explore once the intensity has subsided, and you are left standing amidst the rubble. When you have survived the hardship but feel unclear on where to go from there, this is when the synonymity of Yoga and resilience can, if you choose, help you to move forward from the difficulty and continue to live a beautiful life.

> Grief is the midwife of your capacity to be immensely grateful for being born [Hoffman, "With Memorials," n.p.].
> — Stephen Jenkinson

Introduction
The Myth of Modern Yoga

Yoga is not what you think. It is not what the modern world has turned it into in the last 75 years or more. No matter how much we believe that "Yoga" is what we do on our mat—the stretching, the playlists, the alignment, the posturing, the clothing, the sublime pursuit of light and love, the all-pervading peace—it's just not true, at least not completely. What most people in the West today call "Yoga" is at best a partial truth, a fraction of truth that is incorrectly represented as the whole.

What we do in a "Yoga" class and a "Yoga" studio is closer to pseudo-spiritual physical fitness than Yoga. No more, no less. The reason some practitioners struggle to practice at home can't simply be reduced to the need for classes and community, because it is something else entirely. Because with or without Yoga classes, what we understand Yoga to be might not be Yoga at all. This challenge to our modern belief of Yoga might propel us to defend all the ways that classes and community make us feel more connected, more at peace, calmer, healthier, and happier when we practice. However, these explanations are a far cry from the traditional understanding of Yoga. It's precisely these "reasons" by their very nature that are the proof that what we are practicing is not Yoga. This provocation might seem irreverent, but in fact, it is where true Yoga begins.

What Yoga Is Not

None of the ancient texts on Yoga outline anything remotely related to our modern definition, yet people still believe that this ideal of absolute peace, harmony, and unity is Yoga. Even though not a single text I have read about Yoga, its origin, or its mythology *ever* states implicitly or explicitly that Yoga makes the world a better, more peaceful and loving place, many people believe that is the goal. Even though Yogic text after

5

Introduction

text outlines the challenges, extreme discomfort, difficulties, and often death and destruction that continue to exist despite a Yogic path of practice, our modern view of Yoga holds fast to the achievement of this fantasy of transcendent perfection. The texts on Yoga provide instructions for working with and in difficult situations rather than subverting or transcending them, yet so many modern Yogis continue to believe that "Yoga" will solve all our worldly problems once and for all.

As a teacher of Yoga teachers, I am bombarded with stories of disappointment and disenchantment from students who desired the deeper Yogic education as a panacea for the problems in their families, marriages, jobs, etc., and instead come to have these problems amplified as their practice deepens. Rather than Yoga being a switch that flips your life onto the "good" setting, it lifts the veils of our own ignorance to see what has been there all along, rumbling underneath the surface of our unawareness. This recognition is hard, and it is Yoga.

If we explore the actual teachings of Yoga, we discover that Yoga is quite the opposite of modern-day claims. It is not a practice covered in sticky sweet syrup of positivity. There are no scripted classes, curated playlists, or perfected postures. And while this is understandably disappointing to many modern-day practitioners, this disappointment doesn't cease to make it true. The modern ideas of Yoga, though inaccurate, are a much easier sell to the modern consumer than the truth is. Studios and teachers value what sells, so marketable skills and feel-good products are regularly lauded as Yoga. In rare cases when students sincerely attempt a deeper study of Yoga, the amount of philosophy, self-inquiry, and effort required often leads to frustration and disappointment. The practice of Yoga, which more accurately involves being challenged to think critically and reflect deeply on our contributions to our current life circumstances rather than simply learning rules to follow, is unmooring. Even the invitation to students to question their former beliefs about what Yoga is can cause them to feel angry and disheartened. The idea that the less than celebratory and peaceful feelings that arise through practice are at the root of Yoga can feel defeating, and when the desires for transcendence, peace, and ease that are sold as the product of modern Yoga are exposed as patterns of escape, those excited for Yoga to fix their worldly problems can find themselves thoroughly dismayed.

Our dominant consumerist culture teaches us that the point of the product is to please the customer and that acquisition and perfection make you feel good. "Yoga" then becomes something else to consume. But this is not the true nature or practice of Yoga. Yoga is not now nor has ever been what most modern day "Yogis" think it is, and no amount of argument to the contrary will change that. No amount of validation of personal progress, transcendence, love or light will make Yoga what it is being sold as. Consumers want to feel right, good, and comfortable, but these feelings are not what Yoga is about. When we buy a product that brings attention to our faults, our shortcomings, our imperfections, we will return it because it doesn't work, it didn't give us what we wanted, it didn't make us feel good. If we were told the truth that *Yoga is not designed to make us feel good, to make us feel comfortable, or to support a never-ending quest for success,* no one would want it. The truth is Yoga might just make us feel horrible sometimes. Real Yoga is often the opposite of a feel-good practice because it asks us to become acutely aware of *all* aspects of ourselves, all the pieces and parts that we try so hard not to see, all the uncomfortable, ugly, and abhorrent qualities of our identities. It gathers all the sins and crimes (true or unjustly labeled) to be seen, to be counted, to be included. That is Yoga: bringing the mess of the self into the light of awareness. And our work as Yoga practitioners is to join with it, to yoke to it as true, and then learn how to live with it, how to love not in spite of but because of it all. Yoga teaches us compassion, true compassion, first for us, then for the world.

> Real compassion kicks butt and takes names, and it is not pleasant on certain days. If you are not ready for this fire, then find a new-age, sweetness-and-light, soft-speaking, perpetually smiling teacher, and learn to relabel your ego with spiritual-sounding terms. But stay away from those who practice real compassion, because they will fry your ass, my friend [Wilber, *One Taste*, p. 93].

What Is Yoga?

So, what is Yoga really if it's not the poses, the flows, the music? Let's start with some vocabulary. The word "Yoga" is derived from the Sanskrit root "*yuj*," which means "to yoke" or "join." By the very nature of Yoga, we enter into that from which we feel separate or divided; we don't escape or deny it. The postures we perform in "Yoga" are called "āsana," a word which does *not* mean pose or posture but actually means "seat." In other words, to perform "Yoga āsana," you take a seat in or with what you feel separated from. Another familiar word in the "Yoga" world is "*vinyasa*," which does not translate as flow or the joining of movement and breath but rather means "to place in a certain way." If we practice "Haṭha Yoga," we are joining with every other person that gets on a "Yoga" mat regardless of what style of "Yoga" they are practicing. Haṭha Yoga is simply a category of Yoga that delineates the physical practice from the *rest of Yoga* (which is not the physical practice of āsana). Haṭha Yoga includes *any* style of Yoga that engages in physical practice, meditation, and breathing. One more definition for the purpose of modern Yoga needs to be considered: "prāṇāyāma" does not mean "breathing"; it means the "restraint of the life-force energy." The commonly known breathing techniques of *ujjayi* and *kappalabhati* aren't even technically considered to be prāṇāyāma practices, rather they are *prāṇa shuddhi* practices meant to cleanse and build prāṇa rather than restrain it.

Practices that include the physical movement of āsana (i.e., Yoga poses) are not immediately "Yoga" practices simply because you are practicing Yoga poses. In order for your āsana class to be considered Yoga, even in the strictly physical sense, you would have to practice each āsana as a destination in and of itself rather than use poses to create a physical "flow" of choreography (this practice is more closely linked to dance than Yoga), and you would have to integrate the practices of prāṇāyāma and meditation into the physical practice. Most modern Yoga classes emphasize the physical movement and flow necessary for the achievement of physical fitness and athleticism and altogether reduce or remove the elements of awareness, meditation, and prāṇāyāma that are the essence of Yoga practice.

Yoga Is Inquiry

The real practices of Yoga teach us to inquire relentlessly into the nature of our beliefs. Yoga, when skillfully practiced, results in self accountability and sovereignty. So, if these words and ideas that counter what you have known Yoga to be feel provoking, offensive, wrong, or too critical, then Yoga is the practice that we apply to explore *why* we feel that way rather than immediately judging our experience based on our opinion or the desire to categorize ideas into dichotomies of right and wrong. Though we are taught that to be right is the ultimate achievement, ideas, explanations, and opinions that challenge our ideas of "rightness" do not have to be synonymous with "wrong." The ability to be in the space of conflict and contradiction without dichotomizing the opinions we are receiving is one example of the experience of Yoga.

Yoga Is Exploration

Yoga as a practice is the exploration and inquisition of the self. Yes, that exploration can include but is not limited to the physical experience of Yoga āsana, and it can assess all the ways our bodies are holding patterns of behavior, trauma, or emotion. Physical practice can also include the recognition of our disembodiment or the vacancy and disconnection we have with our form. Yoga also relentlessly applies the skills of inquiry to the mind, including emotion, but does not function like psychology. Instead, it acts as a way to penetrate our identification with our identities and as a tool to challenge us to question it. *Psychologizing is* not *Yoga.* Yoga examines the subtleties of our existence seen through multiple lenses, including but not limited to energy, the elements, the mind, and mythology. Yoga is a practice of attunement, assimilation, and integration bringing together opposing forces into a coherent whole. It hones the tools of concentration and focus. As we practice, Yoga helps us build the skills of staying present in every situation, even and especially the uncomfortable ones, and helps us to probe the truth of every experience rather than fall asleep in our beliefs, our morality, our judgments. Yoga, the practice and the experience, provides us with the agency to be self-responsible and self-accountable in every situation in which we find ourselves. It is an invitation to continually re-orient our attention and to make discerning choices about how we respond. When we live it, Yoga feels like trust; when we practice it, it feels like fire.

So, are we practicing Yoga? Are our *vinyasa* classes inviting us to relentlessly question ourselves, our beliefs, our reactions and experiences (especially the ones in which we feel "right" or "heroic")? Are our studio communities encouraging us to willingly and courageously step into the discomfort and pain of the situations we encounter? Are we living our lives committed to searching for beauty among the mess, jewels among the rubble, joy in the sadness, trust in the fear, expansion in the constriction? Is our practice supporting us in taking responsibility for our contribution to every situation? If the answer is *yes,* then we are Yogis, in the truest form. However, if we find that our practice of "Yoga" looks more like a way to escape the discomfort of our lives rather than meet it, if we find that we need the music to distract us, the heat and movement to "get us out of our minds," if we need our "Yoga" to get back to "normal," then we might *not* be practicing "Yoga," and that's okay. It's a place to start.

Yoga Is a Practice

The true practice of Yoga is synonymous with the lived experience of resilience, and we will talk more about that in the chapters that follow. For now, it's enough to realize that Yoga invites us to start where we are. We

Introduction

can bring the questions, the choices, and the challenges into a space where we become inquisitive. This is a place ripe with the opportunity to learn, to grow, to evolve. Yoga allows us to bring everything with us and to work with what we've got.

Just like all great myths, it's the shiny story of heroes and demons that draws us in. But when we strip away the details, the phantasmagorical accounts, the epic battles, the defeats and the victories, we find, as scholar/ practitioner Douglas Brooks and Yoga teacher Jeanie Manchester say, "we are every character in the story" (Manchester, "The Epic Ramayana," n.p.). We are the multitudinous expression of the whole. The good and the bad coexist within us. The comfort and the discomfort are both expressions of truth. Myths draw us in and give us an encoded map for exploring our inner terrain. So, if the myth you have been committed to is that Yoga is a way to escape or transcend your life, consider this an open invitation to re-evaluate the story. Dare to learn more, to think more critically, to question what you've been told, to interrogate yourself, your feelings, emotions, thoughts, beliefs, and judgments, because this is the practice of Yoga. You are invited right here and right now to begin your practice of Yoga, maybe for the first time, and see what happens.

How We Will Explore Yoga of Resilience in This Book

In the chapters that follow, we will explore Yoga as a powerful tool to assimilate the disparate parts of ourselves into an integrated whole. From this place of wholeness, we will explore how to move through the unrelenting chaos and uncertainty that is life in the world right now. We will dare to be attentive to the parts of the self that we would rather not see and develop a tender sensitivity to the undeveloped and immature aspects of our identity. We will learn how to be in compassionate disagreement with our old and outdated patterns of behavior and how to carry all these skills into the ways we engage with life through relationships and experience.

In this way, we will be using the system of Yoga to support resilient lives. We will explore how to access our strength in the midst of hardship and challenge, how to access wellness without certainty, and how to be responsible for the choices we make. In addition, Yoga and its ally resilience will guide us into the possibility of sustaining fullness and joy in our lives, even though they may fall short of our expectations. Throughout this book, specific techniques of Yoga will be referenced as practices to remember our innate resilience. As the Yoga teacher Erich Schiffmann says, "Yoga is what you practice until Yoga becomes who you are," and I might add that the remembrance of Yoga as our innate state is the experience of resilience itself.

Practice and Application

Each chapter will include a practice section at its completion. The invitation in this section will be to directly apply what you have read and discovered, using the tools of inquiry, movement, and Haṭha Yoga. All the suggestions for what *āsanas* to use and the energetic references found in these sections are expanded upon in greater detail in Chapter 15, "Tools and Supports," in which you will also find explanation, context, and resources for these suggestions.

The tools included in Chapter 15 will support your growing awareness of the subtle yet pervasive power that is the basis of our action and experience. The purpose of the Practice and Application section of each chapter is to learn how to feel, modify, and create energetically specific practices that serve to support your experience of resilience. As such, you will be given opportunities to choose for yourself what practices (*āsanas* and *prāṇāyāma* practices) will best support your current state of feeling and need, and you can refer to Chapter 15 for more specific instructions and guidance. These Practice and Application sections are not meant to be practice plans or scripts, rather they are suggestions as to how the information can be explored and applied through contemplation and embodied movement. Chapter 15 will provide you with the information you need to put together a simple but well-crafted embodiment practice, however you are feeling, wherever you find yourself on any given day. Please refer to it as needed at any point in your reading.

Utilize these steps for the Practice and Application sections:

1. Feel/observe
2. Inquire
3. Assess (movement)
4. Practice/apply (āsana)

Why "Yoga of Resilience" and Not "Yoga for Resilience"

The use of the preposition "of" in the title of this book rather than the preposition "for" is intentional and not to be overlooked. This is not

Introduction

another book of tools and techniques to add to our resilience toolbox. This is not another collection of strategies to apply so that we improve or master the outcome of resilience. This is a book that, I hope, will help us remember that resilience is our marrow; it is the essence at our core. The preposition "for" implies provision, a collection of information, an addition or an offering, whereas the preposition "of" expresses possession, an ownership or property. Throughout this book, I hope to remind us again and again that neither Yoga nor resilience can be learned because we already know it. The application of the practices we find in these pages is meant to help us remember that. Yoga is who we are when we aren't distracted by who we are not, and resilience is the foundation on which we are built. This is a book of returning, not acquiring, and I hope it serves you well.

Practice and Application

Feel and Observe: Take a moment of quiet stillness to observe how your body and breath feel after reading this chapter.

Inquiry: How did this unpacking of Yoga make you feel? Did you sense or feel resistance or defensiveness? Where in your body did you feel what you were reading?

Movement: Follow the body sensations that you discovered and transform them into movement. Do you feel tight in your chest? Can you take a shape or move in a specific way that touches that tension? Do you feel agitated? Jaw clenched? How can you access that sensation through physical movement? Where does it lead you?

Āsana and Energetics Suggestions:

Tadāsana
Uttānāsana
Chakravākāsana
Adho Mukha Śhvānāsana
Sphinx

Focus on feeling your body in these forms. Where do you feel sensation? Where do you feel vacancy or absence of sensation? What movements emerge from the inside of your body rather than from your mind?

1

Resilience Unpacked

"Resilience" is commonly defined as the ability "to withstand or recover quickly from difficult conditions" or the ability "to recoil or spring back into shape after bending, stretching, or being compressed" (Lexico, "Resilient," n.p.). Originally a term used by the science of physics to describe a material's capacity to absorb and release energy and the quality of recovery from the effect of a stressor, the word has been adopted by the field of psychology to describe

> the ability to cope mentally or emotionally with a crisis or to return to pre-crisis status quickly. Resilience exists when the person uses "mental processes and behaviors in promoting personal assets and protecting self from the potential negative effects of stressors" [Wikipedia, "Psychological Resilience," n.p.].

In an increasingly information-saturated world where we are under the stress of exposure on a minute-to-minute basis, it's no wonder that resilience has become the newest cultural pursuit. So many of us are seeking to be more resilient in our family lives, in our professional lives, and in our intimate relationships. So many of us hold the hope that in resilience we will find the peace and ease that we sorely lack. Unfortunately, that is not how resilience works. Being resilient isn't a finish line; it's a state of being, a lifestyle. And it does not result in a more peaceful, less overwhelming life. Resilience is the result of pressure, not the absence of it, and to live resiliently, we must live in and among the chaos and uncertainty of life, rebounding from our troubles, without losing our vitality or enthusiasm.

Resilience Requires Hardship

The hard truth of resilience is that it cannot exist independently of hardship or in denial or rejection of it. Resilience relies on and arises from the hardship itself and is dependent upon the level of discernment we bring to it. In relation to our hardships, resilience isn't something that can be practiced but instead is what emerges naturally as a response to our ability to assimilate, integrate, and grow from our difficult experiences.

Resilience is maturation, which is very different than striving or achieving, and it is most often found in the willingness to surrender to our discomforts and failures. In today's world, we strive not to meet our challenges and accept them but instead to find reprieve, salvation, extraction from difficulties that challenges bring. We endeavor for a life of comfort and security and work hard to contrive situations where we can avoid mistakes, pain, distress, and hardship. This may be precisely why resilience is in short supply. In our attempt to avoid difficulty and pain, our muscle of recovery has atrophied. This also may be why there are so many Yoga classes and practices touting the promised land of resilience as the ability to feel better or rise above our challenging circumstances. Because in truth, most of us would prefer to avoid the pain altogether rather than willingly dig our bootheels into it.

What seems to be conveniently overlooked in the modern practices of resilience is the absolute necessity of our discomfort. Most resilience teachings are about how to be more comfortable or provide relief from our hardship rather than to develop a capacity to sustain and deepen our discomfort. Even the most prominent "Yoga" teachers today promise Yoga can extract you from your difficulties. The Yoga world continues to usurp the truth of resilience and offer instead resilience as a commodity to eject you from your troubles. If you find that no matter how hard you try, you simply cannot escape the obstacles, stress, and pain that life throws your way, perhaps it's time to re-evaluate your approach to mainstream Yoga teachings.

Questions to Explore

The first question to explore is, *"How does resilience feel to you?"* Are you able to identify experiences in which you feel and express resilience in your life? Does resilience feel like calm, peace, letting go? Is it sustainable or fleeting? How are we measuring our resilience as individuals and communities? As a country or a world? Are we calling our desires by the right name, or have we adopted a word that helps us feel more successful and in control and applied it incorrectly to the experiences we are creating? In other words, are our resilience practices really making us more resilient? And how do you know it's working? Though these questions are challenging to the mind and most likely leave you without answers and with more questions, they are necessary, nonetheless.

We can begin our inquiry into our relationship with resilience by wondering about our desired outcomes. Does your practice of resilience actively disassociate you from your discomfort or lead you to explore it? Are you coming to your Yoga mat to slow your breathing, open your body, and feel better or to develop curiosity about your inner experience? If feeling better is the motivation that has you seeking and practicing resilience, a U-turn might be needed. Any practice designed to give us a momentary vacation (disassociation) from our discomforts is *not* a practice of resilience. It is a practice of circumvention.

Instead of strengthening our ability to recover and building the capacity to endure more stress with less detrimental effects, seeking to escape or disconnect from our discomfort might be exacerbating our inability to rebound from difficulty. Though when in a state of trauma or grief, disconnection and dissociation might be necessary for present-moment survival (and these strategies aren't wrong), they are meant to be temporary. When we find ourselves trapped in these cycles of disconnection, we have moved from survival to dysfunction. When we confuse survival strategies with resilience, we often get stuck in unfinished cycles of prolonged suffering. We can unknowingly begin to equate escape with healing. We can find that we keep ending up in repetitive cycles of pain and sorrow rather than moving away from them. We find that we are constantly seeking ways to feel good rather than ways to heal. However, feeling better isn't the goal of resilience, but rather growth, maturity, and feeling *more* are the desired outcomes.

The Relationship Between Resilience and Yoga

Ultimately, neither Yoga nor resilience is something you can *do*. Neither of these practices are something that you can be productive at or achieve. No amount of information and instruction will result in the experience of resilience. Yoga and resilience are what emerge from within you when you let go of the pursuits of success and perfection and when you stop trying to control your environment or outcomes. The primary element of both Yoga and resilience is permission: what is referred to in Yoga as "*surrender*" and in mindfulness as acceptance. When we acquiesce to each moment (every moment) just as it is, Yoga and resilience are what you find waiting for you.

Yoga of Resilience

From a Yogic perspective, this is an invitation to apply the skills that our practice provides: exposure and experience. When we come to our Yoga mat or our meditation cushion, we are entraining our perceptions (thoughts, ideas, judgments, etc.) with our identity (our concept of self). This is what Yogic texts define as "union." To join our ideas, observations, and identifications with our innate understanding is the experience of Yoga. Though simple in concept, this understanding is one of the most complex in application. It is often felt as something like this: In a Yoga posture, like downward-facing dog, there is a physical release, an opening (the hamstrings release and the lower back feels freer and more spacious). At the same time, the mental conflict between the effort to achieve the form and the experience of the form itself resolves. There is a sense that it is not *you* doing the pose but rather you are expressing yourself as the pose. Your idea of what the form should be and the experience of you in the form have merged into a single experience, resulting in the felt sense of you *as* the form. Eventually, even the attachment to the expression/identification of the form dissipates, and you are simply "in" the actions, feelings, and experiences. You are not just the actor but also the action and that which is acted upon.

This felt sense experience is also an expression of resilience. We are no longer battling the onslaught of stimuli or trying to manage, control, or diffuse the chaos or difficulties. Instead, we are recognizing ourselves as an integral but ultimately non-essential part of it all and engaging as such. The resistance to the experience lessens, and the ability to operate within it increases.

This example might stretch the scope of what you currently know Yoga to be, but the teachings of Yoga have been guiding us in this direction for a long time. One of the most foundational (though not beginner) texts of Yoga is *The Yoga Sūtra of Patañjali*. This few-thousand-year-old text outlines the basic understandings of Yoga. It is one of the most popular philosophical texts taught to Yoga teachers in training today, but the modern interpretation rarely conveys the message and intent that Patanjali expressed. In the text, Patanjali teaches that there are three ways to approach Yoga.

1. The mild path abides by the eight limbs (*Aṣhṭāṅga*) and is the path for those who have forgotten who they are as they traverse the journey of life. This path is externally directed for those who have not yet remembered how to hear their internal guidance and feel unable to be self-directed. This path is the most often misrepresented in

modern Yoga teachings. It is presented as a list of "rules" or guidelines to follow in a format familiar to most Judeo-Christian cultures—eight commandments of behavior and expectation. The first two of these eight are further broken down into five additional rules of restraints (*Yama*) and observations (*Niyama*). This path is considered the least risky and is meant for those who do not have a natural proclivity to the intensity of Yoga.

2. The medium path consists of the last three *niyamas* (the second set of the eight limbs) only. This is also known as the path of Kriya Yoga (the Yoga of action) and is composed of *Tapas, Svādhyāya,* and *Ishvara Praṇidhāna*. (We will return to these terms later in the book as we look into the ways we can assimilate resilience into our lives.) This path is for those who are ready and willing to know themselves and be engaged in the practices of surrender and reuniting with innate understanding. These teachings do not require the adherence to the previous sets of rules that Patanjali presents and rather are meant for those who are ready to jump into the necessary risks and challenges of knowing themselves fully. This path requires courage and determination but is free from expectation.

3. The severe path has only two directives: *Abhyāsa* and *Vairāgya,* that is practice and non-attachment (surrender), respectively. Show up in full awareness that you are Yoga being made manifest in the world, then surrender whatever rewards or consequences that you obtain as insignificant to your path. This path is considered the most intense to live and cultivate. It is *not* a path of absence of choice but rather is an invitation to live within the intensity of life's moments, both joyful and sorrowful and everywhere in between, with full awareness of yourself and your role in the experience. It calls for complete engagement and total nonattachment to the outcome. It demands a trust in the self that eclipses the details of the external environment and a clear understanding of the contribution to the whole that one makes with every choice. This is a path of ultimate responsibility and accountability and requires unparalleled bravery, willpower, awareness, and discernment.

The gift of the Yoga sutras is that we are free to choose which path is for us. We hold the power to discern for ourselves which approach works best for us at any given moment without judgment or expectation. If we don't feel ready to lead ourselves into liberation, then we can follow the "rules" as laid out in the mild, eight-limbed path of Rāja *(Aṣṭāṅga)* Yoga (especially the commandments of *Yama and Niyama*). If we feel ready to be self-guided, i.e., responsible and accountable, then we can work the medium path, including all the *Māyā* (illusion/magic) that we carry in order to craft an identity in the world and begin to integrate all the misunderstandings into a cohesive whole. Or we can jump off the cliff of the severe path and be Yoga (fully integrated whole) and release all attachment to security, effort, and achievement.

We are at a crossroads where we have the opportunity to choose how we meet our experience. We cannot control the environment, the circumstances, or the outcome. We can only choose how we will meet it all, and it's not a one-size-fits-all experience. It's a moment-to-moment practice of assessment and response. This is Yoga in practice. This is where resilience can be cultivated. In "this-or-that" moments, we can remember the infinite opportunities that fill the invisible space between the two choices. We can slow down and feel, we can identify our habits and patterns of protection and reaction, we can be gentle and forgiving with ourselves, and proactive in our engagement. We can set boundaries *not* as a means to separate but as an opportunity to re-calibrate and re-align with the knowingness (what Yoga calls *Dhī*) that is perpetually whispering inside of all of us.

Perhaps the best (and hardest) thing we can do is to drop any resistance, judgment, and impatience. To stay present, be with ourselves, be with what is, find gratitude in the seemingly insignificant, and find freedom in releasing control: these are the experiences of the Yoga of resilience. There is much healing to be accessed in the spaces between taking sides, as I will address more in the following chapters. When we take responsibility for our feelings, as they are uniquely ours, we cease to demand our external circumstances to change. When we need to be alone, we can be alone. When we need to reach out, we can reach out. When we need to cry, we can cry. When we need to dance, we can dance. When we are able to attune to our needs, assess our reactions, and engage in a responsive way, we are a living example of Yoga, and we are living the experience of resilience.

To practice Yoga is to be fully alive and have a relationship with all parts of ourselves. That is the unity we seek. To be resilient is to arrive whole and alive in the midst of hardship and challenge, to take down the bricks of protection and projection and be vulnerable (and malleable), to be open to being changed by a situation, and to relinquish control. We learn how to stay aware of the old patterns of insecurity, protection, and expectation that creep in when we aren't looking, and rather than meet these patterns with rejection, we create space to allow and understand them. Resilience doesn't mean we have to be okay or in agreement, but it does mean that we are responsible and aware of however we are, and we use the tools of discernment available to work in the places where we find ourselves. The point isn't to survive or succeed, the point is simply and powerfully to *live*. To be alive in every moment regardless of where that moment leads us. That is Yoga. That is resilience. And it is present in *all* of us.

Yoga and resilience require full *acceptance and integration of* what is.

Practice and Application

Feel and Observe: From a place of stillness, observe the rhythm, depth, and texture of your breath. Does it change naturally as you watch, or does it stay the same? Can you locate from where in your body the breath seems to emerge and return? Is it in your chest? Your sternum? Your diaphragm? Or someplace different?

Inquiry: How did you define Yoga before reading this book? What questions or reflections have been provoked? What Yogic path (mild, medium, or severe) do you explore? How does that translate to other areas of your life?

Movement: Lie down on your back on a comfortable surface. Locate your breath in your body. Allow your body to move with your breath. Press down through the back of your body, bend your knees, stretch your arms overhead, lengthen, twist, curl, unfurl. Move in whatever way you feel inspired to explore as initiated by the rhythm, depth, and texture of your breath. Move in a way that brings more expansion to the points of emergence on inhale and more release to these points on exhale. Allow your body to take whatever shape or form it needs to explore the breath in this way.

Āsana and Energetics Suggestions:
Explore your āsanas as a method of release and relaxation (apāna).

Constructive Rest Pose (CRP)
Baddha Koṇāsana
Upaviṣṭa Koṇasana
Utkatāsana
Tadāsana
Śhavāsana

2

Stress and Resilience

In our modern culture, "stress" has become a buzz word that expresses an experience that must be avoided, corrected, or remedied and has created a populace that values stress avoidance and a litany of management and balancing behaviors that never seem to get us where we are trying to go. In the Yoga world, so many people are finding their way into studios and onto their mats as a result or consequence of stress. Classes, books, workshops, and retreats populate the media, guaranteeing an escape from stress, a reduction of stress, or a healing from it. The result has been that our culture has a fundamental misunderstanding of stress, its expressions, and its requirement for resilience. We find ourselves woefully underequipped to handle stressful situations and often feel victimized when our ideas of a "stress-free" life are derailed.

Defining Stress

So, let's take a look at the relationship between stress and resilience. The origin of the word "stress" is "hardship, adversity, force, pressure" (Online Etymology Dictionary, "Stress," n.p.), and the use of the term in relation to our psychology dates only to around 1955. "Stress," as defined in the field of psychiatry, can fall under the categories of positive stress and negative stress. What's interesting about stress as it pertains to resilience is this: Stress is *required* for resilience. We cannot generate a resilient response without it. In a culture that demonizes stress by identifying it as something to be avoided or, at the very least, perpetually reduced, it's no wonder that our societal and individual resilience is extremely low. We are curating non-resilient lives through our efforts to avoid stress, and it shows.

According to the National Institute of Mental Health ("I'm So Stressed," n.p.), stress is how the brain and body respond to any demand. The "stress response" initiates a complex reaction of mental and hormonal processes that result in a shift of our biological function centered in the autonomic nervous system. When the stress response is triggered, chemical reactions take place to prepare the body to respond in a few primary ways: heart rate accelerates, respiration rate increases, muscle tension increases, and digestion slows down or stops. These physical indicators are often the result of the activation of the classic "fight-or-flight" response, which stimulates the body to spring into action under threat. However, in the last few decades, a more complex understanding of the autonomic system has emerged, giving greater depth of understanding to the effects of stress in both the long- and short-term experience. An in-depth study of these more complex understandings is beyond the scope of this text, but you can refer to the recommended resources listed in the appendix for more information. Deepening your understanding of stress is highly encouraged, as it is often the misunderstood experience of stress, and its very close cousin trauma, that is the main obstacle to resilience.

This basic overview of stress offers a few important points to remember. Stress can be both good (positive) and bad (negative). The rapid increase in heart and respiration rates and muscle tension can also occur in the presence of a positive stressor, like a promotion, a surprise, or exhilaration. The body's response to these positive stressors is identical to the response to danger, though the felt experience of it is defined differently. In addition, stress is not itself "bad" or "negative." In fact, it's a necessary function of our biological and neurological systems. A healthy stress response is one where the body is able to return to homeostasis quickly after an acute stress trigger. This means that small bursts of stress are normal, but the impaired ability to return to homeostasis is where stress becomes chronic and unhealthy. In fact, stress is necessary for the health of the entire system and is the main factor in building and expressing resilience.

Differences Between Stress and Trauma

Stress is differentiated from trauma in modern psychology. Since we are Yogis and not psychologists, the focus of this book is on the relationship between resilience and Yoga and how it relates to stress. However, for the purposes of clarification, it is helpful to take a moment to explore the difference between stress and trauma to support our understanding of resilience. "Trauma" is a person's emotional response to an intensely distressing experience. Unlike ordinary stress and hardships, traumatic events tend to be sudden and unpredictable, involve a serious threat to life—like bodily injury or death, whether real or perceived, and feel beyond a person's control. Most importantly, events are traumatic to the degree that they undermine a person's sense of safety in the world and create an impression that catastrophe could strike at any time. Trauma has five primary manifestations:

1. "Acute trauma" reflects intense distress in the immediate aftermath of a one-time event, and the reaction is of short duration.
2. "Chronic trauma" can arise from harmful events that are repeated or prolonged.
3. "Complex trauma" can arise from experiencing repeated or multiple traumatic events from which there is no possibility of escape.
4. "Secondary" or "vicarious trauma" arises from exposure to other people's suffering.
5. "Adverse childhood experiences" (ACE) cover a wide range of difficult situations that children either directly face or witness while growing up, before they have developed effective coping skills.

Dealing with trauma includes complex processes and behaviors that when addressed can result in resilience but also can hamper the individual's ability to live life fully if the strategies used deepen identification with the trauma or avoid the processes of healing. Trauma and its effects are some of the primary obstacles to experiencing a state of Yoga and living a resilient life. We will discuss these points in greater detail in Chapters 10 and 11.

Stress Avoidance

When the going gets tough, the people go to Yoga. Under the broad umbrella of self-care, humans are finding their way to downward-facing dog, chanting "Om Namah Shivaya," and listening to Yoga teachers expound upon platitudes, such as "the only constant is change" and "let your thoughts float across the blue sky of your mind like clouds." All the while, not unlike Western psychology, the "fix" is only as sustainable as the class itself, and the people that came to class for peace are walking out of the studio fuming in aggravation about the text message received during class, the dishes that aren't done, or the difficulties in their relationship, profession, etc. "Yoga" as an island of peace and harmony that teachers and studios claim rarely endures beyond the āsana class or studio walls, where it is often presented as a way to transcend the real problems of life. Modern āsana classes are avoidance machines and have little staying power when the going gets tough. The chemical cocktail of endorphins from physical exertion, dopamine from a high-energy playlist, and mental influence from a performatively calm and together Yoga teacher have many students convinced of the necessity of their Yoga class to handle their stressful lives, but rarely do they retain the benefits when the class ends.

What if the attempt to avoid stress is the wrong strategy? This question is what Yoga explores and has taught since long before studios and Yoga mats. Yoga was never supposed to fix or solve your worldly problems. Yoga cannot eliminate the stress from your life. Why? Because that is not what *Yoga* does. *Yoga* actually begins when you stop hiding, avoiding, or denying the stressful and uncomfortable aspects of life and start living within them. Resilience is the result of the experience of living within and among our stress. Once we understand the role of stress in resilience and how it relates to Yoga, we can shift our awareness to a conscious understanding of it in the moments when it counts.

Nowhere in the vast compendium of Yogic texts (including those pertaining to āsana) are there promises of peace and bliss attainable simply from a few *chaturangas*, upward-facing dogs, and downward-facing dogs a week. Traditionally, Yoga is not offered as a practice that will eliminate all the stress, challenges, and difficulties from your life. Quite the opposite, actually. The practice and teachings of Yoga tell us that the tools and experiences Yoga offers allow us to stay clear, steady, and responsive in the midst of the turbulence of life. The idea that Yoga is a way to eliminate stress from your life is a fundamental misunderstanding and one of the main obstacles for the practice of Yoga as resilience.

Stress, in its multitude of expressions, is the primary component for resilience, whether that stress is simple and easy to recover from or more complex and spilling into the realm of trauma. Resilience is a response to the many challenges of life that constructs a bridge to joy, gratitude, and even healing. Resilience doesn't require healing in order to be experienced or increased. In fact, resilience is often a precursor to healing, and when accessed, it allows the building and sustaining of the capacity to deal with our difficulties and challenges without losing touch with our aliveness.

Process Versus Product

Modern Yogis view Yoga as a magic pill, a path to peace and harmony, and a mechanism of salvation that can elevate practitioners to a level beyond life's difficulties. And modern Yoga āsana classes claim to be the one-stop shop for all things broken. The truth of the matter isn't as clear and simple, however. *Āsanas* as Yoga postures are the foundation of Yoga in the West, and though they are a very powerful tool in the Yoga toolbox, they are far from the most effective. The movements and breath flood the body with the same feel-good chemicals as a good workout, and if you practice with a very skillful teacher, they may even begin to scratch the surface of the experience of Yoga directly. However, the results of even the most skillful āsana practice are far from cures for the myriad ails that bring students to the mat. As one of my teachers used to say, "there are plenty of advanced āsana practitioners who are also unhealthy assholes."

Take me, for example. I discovered Yoga in my late teens and did very little to adapt my lifestyle while practicing. By the time I was in my early twenties, I was attending six to eight Yoga classes a week, often hungover (and sometimes still inebriated) from the previous night at the bar. I could do amazing things with my body. I could stand in a wide-legged forward fold, grab my right ankle with my left hand, rotate my spine to turn my chest upwards, and grab my left ankle with my right hand from behind my back, but I was still going out more nights than not and drinking in excess. Āsana alone did not turn me into a more mature and measured person, it did not free me from my vices, and it did not solve my day-to-day problems, but it was a gateway into the deeper and more profound practices that have supported me in making lasting and sustainable life changes.

The tool of Yoga āsana is most powerful when practiced as originally intended—as an invitation into self-reflection and inquiry and, therefore, a tool for living a more resilient life. Recall from the introduction that āsana does *not* mean pose or posture but is literally translated as "seat." In a literal sense, the word "āsana" means "seat," as in a chair or seated position. In a functional sense, the word means "to sit with" or "to sit in." So, the function of the forms and postures of Yoga is invitational. Moving our bodies into certain shapes and then bringing our conscious awareness to the experience along with our intentional breath create the experience of sitting with ourselves in specific shapes and often with significant challenge. The practice then provides an opportunity to truly feel what we are feeling rather than to correct or escape it.

Āsana done in this way is centered not around the outcome or production of an advanced shape, but rather it is an opportunity to be directly within the process of self-discovery. Though many āsana classes are focused on the perfect alignment and production of a masterful expression of a pose, the experience of Yoga does not require or even request this perfection. The process of encountering your individual imbalances and idiosyncrasies is an education of awareness, one which builds a bridge into the depths of self-knowledge. When the physical experience results in self-recognition that exceeds that physical expression, then āsana is being utilized as a tool rather than an achievement. This approach to āsana as a way to unfold the experience of Yoga is very slow. Because our modern minds move at warp speed through all our habitual patterns of distraction and dissociation that so often keep us at arm's length from feeling our actual experiences, practicing āsana as a process of sitting with/in ourselves is sometimes an aggravating and laborious shift from what we know, and to reap the rewards it offers requires patience and time.

This is one of the primary teachings of Patanjali's Sutra of which most modern Yoga students are unaware. Yoga is to be attended to for a long time, without break, and with reverence (Sutra 1.14). Though in our "busy" modern lives, we like to equate this instruction with going to Yoga class regularly, it actually means something quite different. The experience of Yoga (i.e., sitting with yourself in the form or shape you have taken) requires a slowing down, a gathering and holding of attention, a willingness to *stay* where you are within all the surfacing feelings, emotions, and experiences, and to arrive respectfully in a way that honors whatever arises, including your discomforts, your emotions, your resistances and tensions.

When we shift our practice from an orientation of achievement (the pose) to a process of experience (āsana), then our physical practice of Yoga has the opportunity to become our very own experience of resilience. With time, we become skillful at meeting ourselves in our discomfort and choosing to stay in it. As we become more able to hold spaces of challenge not simply for the results of physical proficiency but also as opportunities to accept and integrate our constraints into the bigger picture of our lives, we discover our resilience both on and off the mat.

Practice and Application

Feel and Observe: Take a simple shape or āsana, one with which you are familiar and comfortable (such as downward-facing dog or a simple lying twist). Observe how it feels to be present in this shape without including it as a part of a larger sequence. Feel what rises up and calls for your attention as you stay in this form. Take note of not only the physical sensations but also the emotions and thoughts that surface.

Inquiry: What is your relationship with stress? How do you feel it in your body? How do you express it to others? How does it affect your life?

Movement: Allow yourself to move through a series of poses or shapes and become curious about the places in your body where you feel tension. Do you equate this tension with stress? Move in a way that guides the tension or stress you discover down toward your feet and out of your body into the floor.

Āsana and Energetics Suggestions:

Explore your āsana as a way to digest your discoveries and release your confusion (apāna/samāna).

CRP
Chakravākāsana
Baddha Koṇāsana
Nāvāsana
Jaṭhara Parivartanāsana
Legs Up the Wall
Śhavāsana

3

Requirements of Resilience

The Identity Challenge

> The differences in talents, intelligence, knowledge are
> negligible in comparison with the identity of the human
> core.... In order to experience this identity it is necessary
> to penetrate from the periphery to the core [*The Art of
> Loving*, p. 44].
>
> —Erick Fromm

Why are some people resilient and others are not? Why can two similar people experience similar traumas but experience very different outcomes? Why does resilience seem to come naturally to some but is so elusive to others? Biologically speaking, we are a species built for resilience, but not every person approaches or understands it in the same way, and not every individual accesses it. Wondering why one person is resilient while another is not is a complex and interesting speculation, which dovetails seamlessly with the explorations and practices that Yoga offers. Understanding and exploring our identity help us to understand more about why resilience is or isn't available to us and open new pathways of access to a more resilient life.

Who are you? How do you identify yourself? When asked these questions, it's normal to begin our answers by starting from the outside in. We reference ourselves in relationship to our family (I am a mom, a wife, a friend), our professions (I am a teacher, a builder, a farmer), and our hobbies and even passions (I am an activist, a painter, a writer). The biggest challenge is to understand who we are from the inside out, recognizing that all these external relationships are the result of internal character(s) that drives our choices and connections.

Resistance as an Obstacle to Resilience

To understand resilience, we must take more than a few moments to talk about the relationship between "truth" and its foundational support system, perspective. In mid-century psychology, researchers began exploring the impact of cognitive bias on our basic decision-making skills relative to the resources available. They "investigated how people make decisions given limited resources" and how "as a result of these limited resources, people are forced to rely on heuristics, or quick mental shortcuts, to help make their decisions" (Ruhl, "What Is Cognitive Bias?" n.p.). These shortcuts and general rules are ways that our minds are able to quickly and efficiently sort information in order to make decisions, and they have their roots in time, culture, place, and family of origin (all external factors). As strategies for safety and quick decision making, these mental adaptations are useful though limited and often flawed, but they are often inadequate and even damaging when they are left unexamined, forming what is known as "confirmation bias"; "the tendency to interpret new information as confirmation of your preexisting beliefs and opinions" (Ruhl, "What Is Cognitive Bias?" n.p.). From a Yogic perspective, confirmation bias helps us explain the tendencies ("*Vāsanā*" in Sanskrit) of our brains to find ways to align and support our existing perspectives ("*Saṃskāra*" in Sanskrit). To expand our faculties to include multiple perspectives and viewpoints is the practice of Yoga, and it works to dismantle our attachment to our limited identity by questioning and renegotiating our cognitive biases (internal work) and redefining our perspective on a much bigger scale. Both cognitive biases and confirmation biases make up the scaffolding and structure of our identity and are major contributors to resisting resilience.

So much of what is seen as a lack of resilience in our modern world is simply an alignment with the dominant perspective of the person having or reflecting on an experience. Depending on the time period, culture, class, and multiple additional factors that influenced our rearing from early infancy to adulthood, the way you see the world is very different from everyone else, even those closest to you. Though the world itself and its expressions often prove to be quite consistent, our experience of those expressions is unique. Based on the factors that influence identity, we often share similar "truths" or perceptions as others in our same cultural class and generational group, but rarely do these diverse groups share an entirely uniform perception of reality. When we wonder how so many people all living on the same rock hurtling through space can share so many common characteristics yet still have such individual interpretations of the exact same events, we must look through the lens of identity and examine how it works to influence our relationship with the world and with others to understand these differences.

The Identity Trap of Modernity

Yogic texts have been guiding us for centuries in the recognition of the difference between identity and "truth." In modern interpretation, this distinction is often influenced by our consumer culture and our relationship to our material circumstances. In Yoga, the identity/ego self is identified with a lowercase "s," and the true, instinctive, inherent, inner, absolute Self is marked with a capital "S." This explanation is confounding and not wholly helpful when trying to understand the ways we identify and engage with our inner and outer worlds. Often, we are not living with integrity because the identity we present to the world does not align with our inner selves. Though we feel that we have succeeded externally when we mitigate our interior disconnection, our experiences of identity often leave us feeling an internal, unnamable void, which results from severing the ties to our inner understanding. In order to meet the expectations of the outer world, we identify ourselves in cultivated ways that support our experiences of external acceptance and approval. The result is that a huge majority of our modern society measures happiness on external scales of material, financial, and professional success rather than alignment with a sense of internal satisfaction or ease. This results in one of the primary crises of our culture: the loneliness and dissatisfaction that come when we finally realize that we have divorced ourselves from our inner truth, often labeled as a multitude of crises (the mid-life crisis, identity crisis, existential crisis, etc.). Unfortunately, many who experience this crisis of identity fail to use it as an invitation to bridge the gaps between their external identity and internal identification. Instead, they double down on the acquisition of material or external comforts as the remedy, ultimately missing the opportunity for the reconciliation of the inner and outer landscape. As the poet David Whyte says:

> One of the great tragedies of our time is the older generation creating communities of second childhood, creating … an environment where they are insulated in hopes that we will not have to speak what has hurt them or offer a bigger gift to society. Where the final hole on the eighteenth green is like a tiny little grave into which the small satisfaction of getting the ball into the hole substitutes for you making a proper departure out of life ["The Edge You Carry with You," n.p.].

In real life, this discrepancy between our external successes and our internal integrity is made evident by a low-rumbling and ever-present dissatisfaction with our life direction and an unspoken doubt about our life's purpose. Countless students over the years have expressed that though they are "successful" as measured by the standards of culture, profession, wealth, and achievement, they feel unfulfilled, unhappy, and even lost. Many people find themselves entering a Yoga class for the first time looking for "more" from life, hoping that the practice (or the teacher) will provide answers to unnamed but persistent questions about the direction their lives have taken. That quiet voice inside that is urging us to explore and question is the same voice that knows that more is available, and that "more" has very little if anything to do with the measurable outcomes of Western success.

Our modern, free-market culture of individualism often reinforces our identity trap by basing the success of our identity on an externalized scale of productivity, performance, and accolades. If you are productive (often translated as "busy"), you are identified as important. If you perform well—i.e., make the grade, get the promotion, receive the award, grow your investments, then you are identified as successful and worthy of further notice. This places acknowledgment of all achievement as judged by sources outside of yourself. Because of this, we feel bound to a system of worth and validation that is completely externalized and cut off from that voice of integrity within. We base our identification on the feedback we receive from our external environment (parents, friends, teachers, colleagues, bosses, etc.) in a never-ending cycle of forced ignorance of our internal condition. In addition, we are living in calamitous times in which we receive validation and a sense of security by identifying with our traumas, our wounds, and our challenges rather than recovering from them. The paradox of this identity struggle is this: humans long to individuate, to be set apart from the crowd, to be seen as unique and separate from the sea of others, while at the same time, longing to be included as a necessary part of the whole, seeking belonging in the very crowd we desire to stand out from. It's an incredibly conflictual existence, being human.

To deal with the conflict of our humanness, we lean into interpretation, reaching toward what is reflected to us from the outside about our value and importance. We make stories based on input, feedback, and a gnawing sense of want. We attach ourselves to the perception that if we work hard enough, we can be worthy enough to be included, essentially orienting our inner value toward those outside of ourselves to determine our "worth." Because we live in a highly systemized society based on binary dichotomies, we unconsciously tether to our own categorical identification as good or bad, right or wrong, a success or failure, etc. We turn toward our cognitive biases to sort ourselves out, and we calibrate toward the confirmation bias of our existing belief systems. Seemingly without our knowledge, the competition of the internal world versus the external world becomes our perpetual and persistent battleground. Yoga (like many therapeutic approaches, spiritual paths, and styles of psychotherapy) strives to heal this separation and helps us remember the wholeness that contains all the individual parts.

Unfortunately, our society has inculcated our dependence upon these external identifications to such a degree that we feel trapped in our identities without reprieve. We have become afraid to wonder whether the cages of identity we find ourselves in are a true representation of who we are. When we feel trapped in the lives we've created, we struggle to see that we are the ones who have locked ourselves away, handing the keys over to society and the dominant paradigm in which we live. We work instead to fortify our cage in order to control the whispers of the Self, longing for expression, which may be deemed unconventional or deviant. We feel judged by the culture and society that view our uniqueness and divergence as threatening or inappropriate, and we spend our quiet hours, our lonely times, our moments of "introspection" adorning the same cage that confines us with reasons not to break out, choosing not to express our inner self to the outer world. We find myriad (and valid) reasons to justify our own entrapment, and we feel estranged from ourselves and the world around us. We argue against our freedom with learned reasoning for our choices, and we make an effort to temper our qualities like being too loud, too shy, too weird, by modifying our behaviors to meet the expectations of others. We strengthen the bars of our identity cage over and over again until we truly believe that the cage is who we are, ultimately all but silencing the small and quiet voice of truth that whispers from inside. It is this voice that the practices of Yoga seek to reclaim and amplify.

We forget that we are, and have always been, more than our losses or gains, more than our bank accounts, IRAs, or health insurance. We forget that inside, we are more than just survivors. Our forgetting is generative. The more time that passes, the more difficult it is to remember and differentiate the part of you that truly expresses your feelings, your fears, your joys from the parts that are performing the expected roles in the external world. Regardless of how much evidence exists that at the end of our days, we won't long for a bigger bank account, a bigger house, more rewards from our profession, or more proof of our perfection, still the modern worldview propels us to stay trapped, unaware, and pursue external improvement.

Though research shows that at the end of our lives, we will long for meaningful relationships, inner awareness, spaces of forgiveness, and more love, more experience, more celebration of the seemingly insignificant moments of our lives, we continue to believe we are unable to change the trajectory of our days, bound to the external expectations and validations that lead us away from the tranquility and joy that we deeply desire. While we often have a quiet inner sense that the external, material world is not fulfilling and that there is more to life than we know, we often find it difficult to engage with that knowledge. Why? Because to participate with ourselves and the world differently, we might have to change our minds, and changing our minds is not only culturally frowned upon, but it is also neurologically and psychologically difficult.

When was the last time changing your mind (even about the little things) was easy? When was the last time you were able to change your course of thought swiftly, even when you knew it was needed and helpful? Whether it is the result of personal choice or response to the request of others, we resist change with all our might, because we cling tightly to the security of our identity even after we've recognized its inaccuracy. Take comfort. It is not a character flaw or an imperfection; it's our wiring.

> [Leon] Festinger's (1957) cognitive dissonance theory suggests that we have an inner drive to hold all our attitudes and behavior in harmony and avoid disharmony (or dissonance). This is known as the principle of cognitive consistency [McLeod, "Cognitive Dissonance," n.p.].

When we adamantly resist changing our minds (often at our own expense), we are seeking cognitive consistency. Beliefs and ideas that are out of alignment with our cognitive consistency often create a great deal of discomfort and "disharmony," so we resist them, even if they are our own. If we have been taught by others that our experiences, expressions, emotions, and opinions are "wrong," we will turn away from our inner impulses and actively engage in forgetting. So, when thoughts, questions, or realizations about our inner experiences surface, we will work to silence them with innumerable strategies, such as doubt, addiction, disassociation, and distraction. We attempt to continue our alignment and agreement with what we've been educated to do because it is how we feel most secure. The human quest for cognitive consistency causes us to be in a constant state of self-denial and refusal, what the Yogis call "*Avidyā*" (ignorance) and the psychologists call "shadows" or "wounds."

When we become aware of these tendencies, we are often inspired to investigate them further. We are compelled to recognize that there are many parts of ourselves that we have hidden away, silenced, or outright exiled, and we begin to muster the courage and strength to retrieve them. This reclamation of the whole of who we are is a reckoning, and it is the primary power of Yoga and resilience. When we agree to turn toward our stories, our pain, our challenges, and our failures as well as our triumphs and successes, we begin to recover the energy that we thought we'd lost. We begin to author a new story that unifies our disparate parts. This new story demands not the elimination of our less-than-appropriate aspects but the inclusion of them. It asks for allowance of our own desires, which we previously silenced in order to perform as expected, and makes space for the grief that comes when we realize how far away we have gotten from who we truly are. This awareness, which is known in Sanskrit as "*Pratyabhijñā*" ("direct knowledge of oneself"; "recognition"), is one of the most challenging aspects of living Yoga. It requires that we move with and as ourselves, including even the most disastrous moments in our storehouse of experiences in our identity. We cease to point exclusively to the external as the cause of our dissatisfaction and difficulty, and we begin to take ownership of the full spectrum of who we are. The outcome of this willingness to include all our pieces in the whole is that we no longer demand the elimination of any part within ourselves. As a result, we cease to require the modification of our external circumstances before we choose to live fully. This process is at the heart of resilience, and it is the experience of living Yoga.

To turn our minds in a new, inclusive direction that has space for all our thoughts and our beliefs can seem unattainable at times. The idea that we can gather all the parts of ourselves into a meaningful and coherent whole feels idealistic and maybe even ridiculous. But the teachings of Yoga say that it is precisely this wholeness (unity) within us that leads to our recognition of the unity of the whole. In addition, when we push at the edges of our perspective, what we often find there are not simply new realizations and radical ideas but also deep, internal, and consistent murmurings that have been ignored into silence. Turning toward that inner state of recollection is called "*Smaraṇa*" in Sanskrit, and it means "remembrance."

The Relationship of Identity and Resilience

Identity, what some schools of thought and philosophy call the ego, has been the grounds of the main battle waged in spiritual pursuits for eons. The Buddhists try to eliminate it, the Yogis to transcend it, the Christians to surrender it. The challenge in all these approaches is that until we truly know who we are, until we dare to look deeply into our own blind spots, we are not able to harness the experience of resilience that is available to us regardless of our history, our wounds, or our traumas. So, instead of daring to truly know ourselves, many of us choose to become the identity that provides us with the most protection and feels the most comfortable because it is the most familiar (not necessarily because it is the best). This cycle keeps us wanting and waiting for a perpetually out-of-reach future when we are fully healed or where the world is safe before we embark on our own path of reconciliation and resilience (and ultimately healing). In today's trauma-informed society, this often looks like the utilization of our trauma and wounds as an identity shield that keeps us from the rebound of resilience requiring others to shoulder the burden of our sensitivity and pain. In turn, this approach reinforces our trauma (and therefore our identification with it) and continues the cycle of identification. Because the external world is fallible and inconsistent, no level of demand or requirement can keep us safe enough to heal and fully integrate wounds.

Our level of identification with our trauma is directly correlated to our ability to address and eventually heal our trauma. The more we identify with it, the harder it is to heal. The harder it is to heal, the more we look toward an externally perfected space or place where we can feel safe. The result is a strategy of living according to a timetable of "when this, then that" that keeps us at a safe distance from our discomforts and from the opportunity to know ourselves. This distance is also what keeps resilience at bay. Resilience is found in the moments in which we find ourselves. It is not dependent upon external perfection, healing of our traumas, or a righting of wrongs. On the contrary, it is best accessed in the world as it is with all its messy and imperfect conditions, in the absence of safety, and without the promise of something better in the future.

> But the complication is that life comes with no trigger warning. Things happen out of the blue. Something happens, and suddenly, with no preparation, you find yourself in the middle of something that you didn't wish to happen. And I think that's why for me, "here" is really important, because that's the space for—when you are in a situation for which nothing has prepared you, to have the language of "here," it is not gentle. It's not even consoling. It just might be part of the truth. And that can be healing, to simply tell part of the truth [Ó Tuama with Tippett, "This Fantastic Argument," n.p.].

Bessel van der Kolk, author of *The Body Keeps the Score*, refers to the necessity of knowing yourself fully in order to be resilient, which is exactly what Yoga has been guiding its practitioners to discover for millennia. When we dare to know ourselves fully, a knowing that includes the reclamation of our less than favorable aspects as well as our impressive ones, we are able to integrate the disjointed pieces of our experience into a congruent system. This provides the ground from which we can dare to live and thereby address the rumblings of truth and longing that exist beneath the surface of our identities.

An Invitation to Unlearn Your Yoga

Were you taught to trust what you know? Do you silence the voice inside in order to follow others? How much time do you spend training and perfecting your education to receive validation from others who claim to know more than you? Does trusting others above yourself free you from personal responsibility and allow you to disperse accountability onto others? Are you putting all of your trust in Yoga practices based on the teachings of someone else? Are you staying within the lines of rules and requirements in your Yoga because someone else told you it was "the right way to do it"? Do you really know what you know? How would you know?

The experience of Yoga is *the experience* of reunion with our innate intelligence, the reunion of the self we show the world with the Self that exists within. Yoga is the reconciliation of *me* with *Me*. We cannot fail at it. We cannot do it wrong. If the Yoga that we are studying says otherwise, it might be time to question it. And it might be time to ask ourselves why we give our own authority away to others who claim to know more than we do about how our practice should look and feel.

Along the path of our maturity and education, most of us were taught to color inside the lines, to follow the rules, to do things correctly as opposed to incorrectly, to get things right not wrong, to succeed and not fail, to listen and do as we are told. In the process, we have lost our inner compass. We separated from (*Viyoga* as opposed to Yoga) the part of ourselves that knows what's right for *us*. We learned to look to outside authority over inner guidance and to perfect our presentation rather than to feel our sensation. Most of us were educated to doubt ourselves and instead to trust others who had our best interests in mind. Many of us received directions to stifle our own creative processes and do what we were told. In order to be "good," we followed the rules. Lamentably, this loyalty to obedience has often robbed us of the ability to think for ourselves, to make mistakes, to get things wrong, to learn from our experiences rather than trust others. Many of us became afraid to be anything other than perfect, and we have come to treat our unique differences as taboo and sinful. Knowingly or not, we hid the voice of our wisdom away somewhere deep down inside and replaced it with the insatiable pursuit of external knowledge.

This model has become the foundation for most of our modern education and has been applied to modern Yoga as well. It was an easy fit. Teachers are given rules to follow, scripts to perform, "right" things to say, "right" ways to say them. Modern Yoga classes and the education of teachers are producing teachers that sound alike, that are uniform, that are predictable (much like the uniformity of individual Starbucks cafés), and lessons that are all but absent of Yoga. Yoga teachers are learning ways to keep students safe at the expense of experiencing Yoga. They are limiting their creativity and asking students to do things the "right" way, enforcing angles and degrees and alignment cues as if all bodies are exactly the same and all desired outcomes identical. Students are discouraged from listening to their inner guidance with exhaustive instructions and external distractions, like flashy playlists and hot rooms. Yoga, contrary to its creative essence, has begun to look like one thing rather than the multitude of expressions it has the capacity to take on. The practice of Yoga has become a practice of coloring inside the lines, following the rules (or limbs), and looking outside the self for guidance.

But what if every "right" experience of Yoga didn't look exactly the same? What if everybody was allowed to be the unique and individual expression of Yoga that they are and not required to mimic a paradigm of the correct or advanced? Are teachers telling students to follow the rules because it's "right" or because they are scared of being "wrong"? What if Yoga was not a vertical climb to success and achievement? What if the real experience of Yoga happens outside of the lines? What if Yoga doesn't have anything to do with the opinions of others and everything to do with the voice of wisdom inside? What if there was no right or wrong in Yoga? What would practice look like? What would teachers teach? How would we know what to do? By courageously turning inward, into the chaos that we want to quiet, into the tension, the resistance, and even the pain that we mistakenly believe Yoga will remedy, we may find that Yoga has the capacity to educate us about ourselves, for ourselves, by ourselves, as ourselves. This approach to Yoga takes courage (*vira*) and a deep connection to your own personal feelings and inner guidance (*bhava*). To dare to make Yoga an experience rather than an achievement, to bravely doubt and question the system of right and wrong, the teachers who inform you, and even the information itself seems to be a path that breaks all the rules. But it might just be the gateway to freedom and most certainly is the way to living resiliently.

Living Resiliently in Modernity

If the upheaval of the last months and years have taught us anything, it's that the things we have depended on are questionable. The ideas of right and wrong, good and bad, happy and sad might not be exactly what we have been told they are. The old systems of success and safety might be illusions, and if we are to be resilient in times of trouble and difficulty, it is up to us. Yet, when so many of us found our dependable structures starting to wobble, rather than feeling set free or capable, we felt rudderless, confused, and unsafe.

Until we become aware that our models of safety are outdated and even false, we will continue to be trapped in our identity cages of success and failure. Though I've told students for years and years that you can't fail at Yoga, both students and teachers in training have consistently refused to believe it. Committed to the systemic model of culture that is the source of our education, students struggle to see Yoga as an experience rather than a requirement or proving ground. You cannot fall short in Yoga; you can simply be where you are, and the same is true for life. Only and always. *We* are the measurement of success, not the achievement of a perfect posture or an advanced technique, not perfect behavior, or supreme success. Wherever we find ourselves is perfect, because we are showing up for what is, as it is. Yoga is more than we realize until we see that Yoga simply is the experience that teaches us to be us, in every moment, in every relationship, in every situation. Yoga is the experience of trusting our inner authority and being aware of our tendency to forget, and it's the experience of remembering. What Yoga, like resilience, asks us to do isn't improve, only to be engaged, awake, and responsive. Yoga doesn't ask for or require perfection. In fact, it thrives on our imperfections, our mistakes, our forgetfulness. Yoga is the experience of clarity beneath the static of input, expectation, demand, and fear. It's always there, even when you forget, even when you can't see it. It never disappears. It is the core of who you are, no matter how you are, where you are, or when you are there.

One of my teachers says, "Yoga is who you are, and you practice to remember that." We are the experts because *no one* can know us as well as we know ourselves, if and when we choose to know. So, though there are myriad techniques for choreographing an āsana practice and there are exhaustive instructions for safety, alignment, and uniformity, none of these tools are Yoga, and the utilization of them doesn't automatically lead us to resilience. If we want to learn how to access the wisdom inside that can guide us to our inner knowing ("*Dhī*" in Sanskrit), then we must be courageous enough to truly know ourselves.

This path of Yoga takes courage; it's the path of the warrior. The Yogi is a hero, and this is the path of resilience. It's full of opportunities to make mistakes and to learn from them. It calls us into direct experience and doesn't provide an all-knowing authority to tell us all the right things to say or do or catch us when we fall (or fail). Instead, Yoga teaches us that the source of our knowledge is based on connection, and to be connected is to be resilient. When we cultivate connection to ourselves, our fellow practitioners, our community, and ultimately everyone else, we source strength, capacity, potential, and power. When we dare to allow ourselves to be seen and known, connection is the result, and it is the bedrock of a truly resilient life.

Practice and Application

Feel and Observe: Turn your attention inward. Land inside yourself. How do you feel in this moment? Where is your attention? Feel your sensations as yourself rather than something happening to you.

Inquiry: Who are you when you aren't busy being who you thought you were supposed to be? What does *your* Yoga look like if you release all the rules and directions?

Movement: Be still. Sit or stand or lay down and move your breath into your abdomen. Feel your belly rise on inhale and fall on exhale. Move through the *āsanas* listed below (or whatever shapes your body is calling you to do) while maintaining this focus on your breath in your belly. Allow yourself to linger in each form or shape for a while. Observe the sensations, thoughts, and experiences that arise. Sit with what bubbles up to the surface and recognize it all as part of yourself.

Āsana and Energetics Suggestions:
Explore your āsanas *as a way to assimilate what you are discovering about yourself* (samāna*).*

Tadāsana
Utkatāsana
Parivṛtta Pārshvakoṇāsana

3. Requirements of Resilience

Nāvāsana
Śhalabhāsana
Ardha Matsyendrāsana
Bālāsana
Śhavāsana

4

Resilience Requires Connection

I live my life in widening circles
that reach out across the world
["Widening Circles," n.p.].
—Rainer Maria Rilke

According to author and neuropsychologist Rick Hanson, every human being has three basic needs: safety, satisfaction, and connection. And we meet these needs in four primary ways: recognizing what's true, resourcing ourselves, regulating our responses and emotions, and relating to others. In order for us to be resilient in life, others are a requirement. In the practice of Yoga, the necessities of connection, relationship, and community are often misunderstood and bypassed for the singular pursuit of unification, commonly expressed as "oneness." However, what Yoga says about connection and oneness is quite different than the way it is commonly pursued today. Yoga as connection is not a transcendent space but an immanent one that requires others and all their unique expressions in order for any individual to thrive. This difference is important for understanding how Yoga and resilience are synonymous rather than disparate paths of pursuit.

The word "Yoga" does not mean "union" as commonly interpreted in the West. The word is derived from the Sanskrit stem "*yuj*," which means "to yoke" or "join." In other words, it means to connect two (or more) things so they can move together. Yoga in practice and experience is closer to calibration and reconciliation than union. It is understood in Yoga that whether or not you believe your physical, manifest, incarnate form is part of something bigger, you are living within this individual form that is in itself inseparable from the illusion of separateness. That you are not your brother, your mother, or your neighbor is understood. Rather, you are a distinct and individuated piece of something bigger than you. Therefore, it's the pieces that make up the whole that are emphasized in Yoga, not the absence of them. So, if Yoga's goal isn't the reduction of the individual into a single unified whole, how can we clarify our understanding of what Yoga is in order to unfold the experience of resilience?

To begin, we must move from striving to return to a state of grace and toward the recognition that we are living within a graceful state with the tools necessary for our aliveness all around us. When we recover this understanding, we can begin to comprehend how and why connection is essential for our experience of Yoga and our expression of resilience.

The reconciliation of our separateness (*Yoga*) is quite different from the dictionary definition of unity: "An undivided or unbroken completeness or totality with nothing wanting; the quality of being united into one" (WordNet, "Unity," n.p.). This common misinterpretation often leads Yoga practitioners away from the experience of resilience rather than toward it. When the practitioner makes unbrokenness, absence of want, and oneness the goal, the opportunity to view the messy, hard, and often disappointing aspects of life as essential parts of the whole is often lost. To find the Yoga that is synonymous with resilience, the recognition of our separation and our technicolored experience is necessary. Through this acknowledgment, it is possible to discover the points of convergence where we are at once very distinct from each other as well as undeniably the same. This experience is the foundation of empathy and the primary threshold of connection. It is a process of reconciliation that allows us to retain both our separateness and cultivate our connection in ways that support our boundaries and express our resilience.

Connection

I often express to my Yoga students that Yoga is a solo practice, but you can't do it alone. This may sound like a riddle, but it's actually the key to understanding why connection is essential to both the practice of Yoga and the experience of resilience. Both Yoga and resilience are experiences of a deeply personal and individual nature. To be truly experienced, they cannot be defined by a set of rules or a standard to follow. Both require reflection, internally and externally, as well as offer the opportunity to communicate and connect about what is expressed and shared. Expression and sharing bring our personal, private experiences out into the world for others to engage with, and this means we must dare to be vulnerable, courageous, and trusting. These very same qualities are inseparable from true connection. They are required for resilience to be accessed and retained. We cannot bring ourselves to the depth of relationship alone, even if the relationship is with ourselves. In attempting to do so we often undermine the very experience we were seeking.

Community

In Buddhism, the teaching of the Three Jewels instructs practitioners to take refuge in three things. To understand the instruction, we must begin with the idea of refuge. Taking refuge (or what one of my teachers, Bayo Akomolafe, calls taking sanctuary) is to meet the irrefutable need for the life raft of resilience. And the guidance for where to find this raft is within the Three Jewels themselves. Buddhist practitioners take refuge (a safe place; a shelter from danger or hardship; act of turning to for assistance) in order to have the necessary resources to sustain the hardship of living and keeping aliveness present. The Three Jewels in which refuge is sought are the Dharma (teachings), the Buddha (teacher), and the Sangha (community). In this teaching, the necessity for connection is essential to resilience and supports the more internal spiritual work. Understanding this helps us to recognize how community is important for our individual pursuits, and how how individual work supports our communities.

I am not qualified to speak on Buddhism, but the idea of a sangha is essential in Yoga as well. "*Sangha*" is a Sanskrit word that means "association, assembly, company, or community" and is an integral part of spiritual practice. Often referenced as a community of like-minded practitioners, a sangha creates a structure in which you navigate the choppy waters of self-understanding among others on a similar path. The members of your sangha provide the feedback, reflection, and understanding necessary to uncover the hidden parts of the inner landscape that are playing a part in keeping resilience (and Yoga) at bay.

Contrary to the modern expression of sangha, the community of care is more than simply a cheerleading squad to support every idea, thought, or realization. Rather, it is a deeply loving, caring, acknowledging collection of fellow practitioners, friends, and intimates who comprehend the value of self-recognition as essential for the health of the entire community and beyond. Often healthy community support involves challenging our ideologies and beliefs, questioning our motivations, and compassionately disagreeing with our views in order to lead us into deeper levels of reflection. In this way, those that nurture us the best also solicit self-accountability and responsibility as a necessary part of our growth and do not simply cheer us on as we face challenges and difficulties.

Support that doesn't equate to agreement and enabling is often disregarded or even rejected, though it can still include the validation and understanding needed to convey love and support. Though, the absence of agreement can sometimes elicit defensiveness or be viewed as threatening rather than encouraging and caring, how we receive and interpret the feedback and input of others is a marker of what drives us in our engagement with the world. We evidence what we want and what we value in the kinds of relationships and support we seek. Without awareness, we often perpetuate our difficulties through the relationships that we cultivate.

Connection Versus Codependence

So often, we equate support with being affirmed and having others see things our way. When someone else expresses their agreement with us, essentially confirming our "rightness," we equate this with connection. We desire agreement with our choices and behaviors and feel "safe and supported" only when we are validated by others. Conversely, we can feel threatened and unsafe when our choices meet dissent, especially from those that are closest to us. This distinction is important in understanding the difference between codependency and connection. Codependence requires enabling, and connection resists it.

Emerging in the distinction between connection and codependence is an interesting paradox: what we perceive we need to feel "safe" only exacerbates our feeling of insecurity (or in this case externalizes it), leaving us feeling dependent on the source of validation as our touchstone to safety, which causes causing us to feel less and less confident in our own internal sense of trust and security. In other words, what makes you think you are safe is often your primary source of insecurity, and what makes you feel insecure can be the experience that leads you to the greatest security. This is the muck that we must wade through to fully understand how and why those that seem to have our best interests in mind, that celebrate us with the most vehemence, are often the very obstacles to our growth.

True and supportive connection does not equate with only agreement and affirmation. Instead, it calls for our connections to be accepting and allowing of who we are without requiring us to change our opinions or behaviors (even if change is in our best interest), all the while being an ally on the path of our growth and self-awareness. Evidenced through the compassionate confrontation of our misunderstandings and the courage to shine a light on our blind spots, these types of relationships are only supportive to those who are ready to participate in them ("*adhikara*," meaning "qualification" in Sanskrit) and often feel as challenging as they do caring.

Steeped in our misunderstanding of agreement as the proof of connection, it's easy to feel that we must sacrifice our beliefs and desires in order to maintain connections based on consensus and approval. This misunderstanding is one of the primary difficulties in accessing the experience of resilience and Yoga. This type of connection leads us further away from the truth of who we are and is reinforced by the idea that true love and support is the result of self-sacrifice and serving others above ourselves. Connection in this way is tenuous. It keeps us dependent upon and constantly vigilant for the approval of others and assumes the need for adaptation and adjustment of our behaviors as the requirement for acceptance and belonging. As patterns of dependent and enabling behaviors compound, we work harder and harder to hide our own desires and longings away in the service of others. The more we hide ourselves away, the farther we are from achieving integrity, and this is the quicksand of enabling and codependency. The result is often resentment, resistance, passivity, and aggression. Our disconnection from ourselves is blamed on others, and we find ourselves at their mercy, helpless to change ourselves.

In codependency, we place requirements on others to complete our story, to change our circumstances, and to meet our needs. Necessitating others' choices and experiences as the source of our own happiness leads us to disconnect from our own desires, though they do not cease to exist. We hold to these patterns of self-sacrifice as a requirement of continuing the connection and depend on others' actions to be the source of our happiness and fulfillment: a losing game that can never be won by any player involved.

The alternative is to be anchored in true support that is cultivated internally and is completely in line with our personal desires. This type of support engages boundaries that orient our understanding intrinsically, reminding us that true knowing is contained within us and is not predicated on the validation or approval of others. When we turn inward for our guidance and respond to that guidance with our outer actions, we seek connections that invite us to embrace and respect ourselves. We strive to show up in our relationships as fully responsible and accountable for what we bring and in doing so, liberate others from the need to make us happy, safe, or understood. We recognize that clinging to unhealthy convictions which demand us to disregard our boundaries and desires is problematic for everyone involved, including for those that we perceive we are helping.

We become aware that holding on too tightly to anyone limits their happiness as well as our own. We begin to acknowledge and respect our own needs, allowing all involved to pursue their unique experience of alignment with integrity and joy.

For those that are enmeshed in relationships of codependency, this liberation can be terrifying and overwhelming, and without a doubt, the risks of change and challenge are high. When our role in our relationships has been the same for a long time (maybe years or even decades), there is a risk that reorienting our behavior toward the cultivation of integrity by aligning ourselves with our inner understanding and autonomy might be uncomfortable for others. If you have been the quiet, accepting friend who has bitten your tongue for 20 years and suddenly you dare to speak your feelings and opinions even when they are different than your friend's, you risk rocking the boat of a long-term friendship. But Yoga and resilience would say the risk is worth the reward. Ultimately, when we disentangle ourselves from our codependent relationships, we also disentangle ourselves from the safety of the familiar. Stepping willingly into the discomfort of the unknown can set us free to explore possibilities of support, respect, and engagement that we weren't able to consider before.

Challenge and Safety

Resilience requires growth, expansion, and discomfort. Yoga teaches us to stretch our perception of what is fixed and static by pushing against the sharp edges of our limits then daring us to sustain the discomfort of unknown possibilities. From this view, our connections can both support us and be our obstacles to resilience. When we stop confusing consensus for connection, we can renegotiate our agreements of reassurance and safety by becoming willing to explore and question the status quo. We allow ourselves to wonder about ideas like: Is it true that love and connection must be expressed exclusively as agreement and compliance? Can we expand what's possible in our existing relationships as well as be open to new supportive connections?

Inquiry and curiosity build healthier relationships that make space for our wants, our desires, our truths, and even our shadows In allowing this for ourselves, we make space for the wants and desires of others. We become our own stable foundation and discover space to receive feedback from those that are closest to us without defending against their opinions.

We begin to see the kernels of truth and growth that are available from others' observations. In truth, many of the most powerful and transformative connections call on us to recognize our unseen parts and require us to review our understanding of safety and threat, ultimately growing our capacity to endure and thrive. As we recognize the resistance to challenge and the requirements of safety as our main obstacles to resilience, we recalibrate our connections from those that feel safe and familiar (and therefore do not challenge us to grow beyond our own illusions) to those that push the edges of our perception and allow us to grow more than we ever thought possible.

In my own life and practice, I find this level of connection both challenging and immensely rewarding. My logical and analytical mind is well developed, and I love a good mental joust. I enjoy debate and the intensity of countering one opinion with another. I enjoy provoking thought and inquiry. It is easy in these circumstances to convey my opinion as the right one in opposition to the opinion that I am attempting to counter, therefore making my counterpart wrong. But that approach often leads to disconnection, hurt, and shut down. Over the years, I've learned how to share my own feelings without the need to convince others and recognize that my feelings are not the only ones that exist. I've learned how to engage in inquiry of my own opinions as well as others and to explore the questions that are offered. When I speak in ways that create space for the opinions and beliefs of all involved my understanding grows and so does my connection with my companions. This connection builds trust so that everyone feels they can share their opinions, and ultimately everyone involved feels included, seen, heard, and valued. The challenge still exists, but the outcome is one of confluence rather than contrast.

The power of connection is in its paradoxical nature. The most impactful and transformational connections provide the experiences of both challenge and safety. The result, is a gateway to resilience. If we are unaccustomed or resistant to personal self-reflection and feel unwilling to do the work of knowing ourselves beyond the familiar identities we have crafted (both consciously and unconsciously), then it can happen that we attract certain connections in order to perpetuate our identity, our comfort, our familiarity, and our inertia. These connections become uncomfortable in their own right by reflecting back to us the things we don't desire to see in ourselves. If we find ourselves in the same unhealthy and dysfunctional relationships again and again, from a Yogic perspective, this is evidence that we have not done the powerful and necessary inner work of self-reflection. If we have not applied the tools necessary to integrate

46

our understanding, then we have not yet digested the experiences that feel familiar yet continue to keep us stuck in the patterns of difficulty that we translate as safety.

How can our connections support our growth and resilience? Supportive connections allow us to develop a deeper capacity for challenge as well as provide nurturance, compassion, and empathy for our struggles. A practice of getting to know ourselves opens the space for healthier and more supportive connections, and there are three steps we can use as we embark upon the process: (1) attenuate, (2) assimilate, and (3) integrate.

Attenuation

"Attenuation" means "to lessen the amount, force, or value of; to make less complex; to weaken." When we attenuate our discomforts and difficulties, we turn toward ourselves in search of the source of our pain. We allow the experience to be felt, and in doing so, we reduce the power that the discomfort has over us. This requires us to slow our minds enough to feel connected to the experience that we would have habitually avoided or denied in our past. In practicing attenuation, we strive to hear what is being said, to feel what arises, to allow ourselves to be present with the uncomfortable. Attenuation requires that we make space to understand our feelings as they are (regardless of how they were initiated) without attempting to fix, change, alter, or adapt them. With practice, attenuation can take a relatively short time though initially it may a while to get started. It requires the willingness to show up with our less-than-optimal feelings, as well as the willingness to receive the critique of others. It may take days, weeks, or even months of continually reminding ourselves to turn inward to seek the source of our discomfort rather than outward to blame or projection.

With practice, attenuation helps to soften the sharp edges of judgment, criticism, and reproach and aids our transition into connection and understanding (this is also understood as empathy). In time, we learn how to be present with our internal disagreements and difficulties and, in turn, to translate them as an opportunity to expand ourselves. Our personal discoveries extend into an understanding of others and help to build new patterns that grow our emotional intelligence and feelings of security within unfamiliar places.

It takes determination to do the work of attenuation because looking toward the parts of ourselves that we don't like, or that other people can see is terribly uncomfortable business. As a teacher, I receive countless emails full of criticism of my approach and that admonish me for everything from my organizational style to my pedagogy. My inbox is never short of opinions on how I can do better or do more. For years, these words felt like attacks, like knives through my heart. My pulse would quicken, my ire would rise, and the feedback would gnaw at me for days and sometimes weeks or months. When I began to work with the tool of attenuation, the comments continued to feel sharp, but I was able to turn toward the truth that they contained. In each was a kernel of reflection that was authentic and real, places where I could work, refine, and grow. In them I discovered the unspoken pain of those who offered complaints, allowing me to open my heart to more empathy and understanding (even if I didn't agree with the opinions). Attenuation allowed me to soften my personal defense and see the truth of both myself and others cultivating the fertile ground of compassion and understanding for everyone, including myself.

Assimilation

To "assimilate," we "appropriate and transform or incorporate into," a synonym for which is digestion. We take all that we have discovered in our attenuation phase, and we break it down to its constituent parts. We dare to be curious about our discoveries, and we bravely inquire about their origins and effects. As we do, we develop an understanding of our patterns and ourselves. Assimilation is the process of digesting the sustenance of our experiences, breaking down what we have taken in, retaining the nourishment from it, and releasing the toxins and "waste." In a practical sense, this could look like turning toward the intensity of a shameful behavior or reaction and staying with it until the force of the reflection begins to soften (attenuation). Then becoming curious about our actions and behaviors, we can empathize and understand the lessons available and forgive and accept our imperfections (assimilation). From this point, we are ready for the integration phase.

Assimilation in action can look many different ways. One way is recognizing when you are on the precipice of repeating a familiar behavior that you desire to change and choosing to do it differently. A silly but very real example of this in my life is as follows. I am horrible with directions. I often do not know how I survived before the little voice in my phone started informing me of every impending turn, and even still, I often find myself lost or turned around. It is not uncommon for me to take the same wrong turn over and over again, thinking "I got it right this time," only to find that after a mile or two, "I've done it again," and I have to turn around to head in the opposite direction. After making mistakes repetitively (and often without my full attention), I become habituated to that mistake, and its pattern becomes familiar territory. However, when I decide that I don't want to repeat that mistake, I turn toward it and really take in the "wrong" choice. I pull up to the intersection and take a breath, I recall my past experiences, I anchor my attention, and in my mind, I consider all the options.

I take a moment to digest the past mistake fully. In doing this, I realize that the last time I was distracted by thoughts or concerns, I was off in a daydream, or I was lost in a love song, and I recognize that this time I have the chance to do it differently. Then, I choose. In truth, it's a 50-50 chance that I will choose the correct direction, but what is for certain is that the pause, the attenuation, the recollection, the attention helps to ensure that I am less likely to repeat the mistake in the future. Eventually, with enough repetition of the process of assimilation, I rarely, if ever, repeat the wrong turn because I have fully integrated the experience.

Integration

"Integration" is a process of claiming our experience fully and is defined as "making into a whole or making part of a whole." This is Yoga: to take all the individual parts and allow them all to coexist as a harmonious, comprehensive completeness. The process of integration reduces doubt, increases acceptance, and makes space for the whole of who we are to be present and available. It does not attempt to fix or remove our imperfections. Instead, it calls on us to be accountable for each gnarly and lovely part of ourselves and to exercise agency in how we will use all these parts. When I fully assimilate the repetitive mistake of the "wrong" turn, eventually, I just know the right direction to choose. I no longer have to take long pauses to attenuate and assimilate all the past experiences and present-moment information. There will come a time when I simply choose the correct direction, each and every time. The discomfort of doubt in my ability will fade, and I will become confident that each time I come upon the intersection, I will make the "right" choice. I have not forgotten nor do I deny all the times in the past when I chose incorrectly. But I also don't take the same amount of time to contemplate it. Instead, the "right" choice emerges from all the lessons I have learned, and it becomes the new integrated behavior.

When we do the work of integration, we are living Yoga, and we are showing up in all aspects of our lives as resilient, vital, and compassionate human beings. When we learn the power of connection within us first through the processes of attenuation, assimilation, and integration, we are able to move out into the world with a greater capacity to create, support, and sustain healthy connections.

Healthy connections are necessary for resilience. For us to live our lives in ever widening circles as Rilke suggests, to grow our capacity to take in more, to allow for more without expectation or requirement and show up simply for the sake of what we will encounter. This is the essence of what resilience and Yoga offer. We can only know that we don't know, and we can trust that our unknowing connects us all through the threads of time to the potential of expanding beyond what is currently known. This is an opportunity to receive and return the innate vitality of engagement without a fixed set of regulations that must be met. When we become willing to access our life force even in the most challenging of circumstances, we are, in our essence, resilient.

Practice and Application

Feel and Observe: Be still and notice the sensations in your body. Notice the feelings of connection in your body. Feel and observe the connection of the inhale and the exhale. Feel the connective tissue at the joints of your knees and elbows, your hips and shoulders. Observe the quality of connection within your physical form. Now, call forth an image of something outside of yourself from which you feel disconnected. Observe the feelings that arise when you think on it; observe the sensations and breath.

Inquiry: What arises when you call up a past experience of pain or discomfort? Can you turn toward your role in the pain that you feel? Can you become aware of how your actions, responses, or feelings influenced the situation? How did you contribute to your own pain?

Movement: Turn on music and close your eyes. A song that pulls on your heartstrings is a good choice. With eyes closed, follow that pull with your movement. Fold in or expand out; move your feet or stretch your arms. Can you make contact with the emotions and sensations within your form and open to their movement? If something begins to feel too intense, you can shake out your hands or feet or even your whole body. Go gently. Don't force it.

4. Resilience Requires Connection

Āsana and Energetics Suggestions:
Explore your āsanas *as a way to circulate your insights and agitations* (vyāna).

Tadāsana
Vīrabhadrāsana II
Trikonāsana
Sphinx
Paschimottānāsana
Śhavāsana

5

Enchantments of Experience

If our experiences of reality are dependent on so many unique factors of identity, will we ever agree or share a common understanding? Yoga says "yes": not by eliminating the factors and experiences of our unique perspectives, but by understanding the map on which they are charted and giving space for the full expanse of the terrain. We've been exploring an array of Yogic thought in the preceding chapters. Now, we will shift to more a more specific exploration of the foundational understandings of Yoga. A note before we begin: the complexities, intersections, juxtapositions, divergences, and contradictions within any given system of Yoga are vast, with each system containing both striking similarities and distinct differences. In an attempt to explore these complexities, I have been drawing from only a handful of the varied Yogic philosophies in the hopes of establishing a greater common understanding of our undoubtedly distinctive human experiences. But by no means does this sliver of information begin to capture the vast scope of philosophy and expression of Yoga.

From a Yogic perspective, all our incredibly diverse and individual experiences can be mapped onto a similar basic premise. That there is something bigger than our incarnate, material human and worldly experience is something on which most, if not all, systems agree. How each system refers to the bigger force is unique and diverse as the expressions of existence themselves, and the relationships and practices related to these expressions are also unique. The belief that humanity (and all the material expressions of worldly existence) is simply part and parcel of something much bigger is not unique to Yoga either. This understanding is reflected in most of the known spiritual systems of the world, the reflection of each being unique to the individual system.

To unravel the multiple threads of understanding of what this inexplicable, non-material mystery is or how it works exceeds my capacity as a student and practitioner of Yoga. So, instead, I work from a foundation of understanding that acknowledges something beyond the corporeal and leave it up to each individual to interpret the what and how for themselves.

52

Understanding Yoga More Deeply

Though many modern Western Yoga "systems" are attempting to neutralize Yoga's core spiritual teachings, it doesn't take too much looking to uncover the deeply profound and mystical concepts underpinning the physical and breathing practices that most modern Yogis associate as Yoga. Let's unpack some of the more esoteric ideas of this spiritual system in order to lay the bedrock of the structure that is synonymous with resilience.

One system that Yoga philosophy draws upon, *Tantra*, states that humans are a microcosm of the macrocosm. In other words, every person is a tiny version of the universe in its entirety. Though this might be a stretch for the mind, it simply states that the clear and defined principles that underlie the universe are the same clear and defined principles that form the basis of our humanness. We are built upon a foundation of fairly straightforward rudiments onto which we pile the unique and multifarious complexities that make us distinct and individual.

I know, at some innate level, that I am different from you. We are not the same. Yet Yoga (and in many ways the experience of resilience) asks us to stretch our sight beyond the concrete separation and dive into the elemental resemblance and correspondence of each other's intrinsic selves.

Contrary to common teachings, Yoga is not attempting to homogenize existence into one uniform experience, but rather it is guiding us to remember that everything is made up of the same thing, and that same thing is mysterious, beyond knowing, and expressing itself in innumerable sentient and non-sentient ways. The combinations and complexities of expression are infinite, but the building blocks are minimal (and irrefutably the same). Here again, I step out of the zone of my expertise, but the point to be made is this: From the sameness, the multitude that we are emerges. From one, come the many. From a Yogic perspective, we the people are the expression of boundless individuation, experience, and combination, and it's this very relationship of simplicity and complexity that makes us beautiful.

Yogic practice is not meant to disregard these unique expressions of self but rather is a system of honoring and celebrating difference as well as remembering (*Smaraṇa*) our innate sameness. This teaching can be viewed through the lens of both the macrocosm (that we are all made of about 60 percent stardust and water, elements of which have been recycled since the beginning of time, expressed in countless combinations from rivers, to oceans, to raindrops, to human bodies) and the microcosm or, in other words, *you*.

I want to emphasize that I do not intend to oversimplify the complexity of our human existence; I merely wish to establish a common ground from which we can begin to explore it. One of the most phenomenal expressions of our complexity is the enchantment of our identity. We have already established a basic understanding of identity, its necessity and its tendency to complicate matters. Now we will begin to look at why this is important and even necessary, according to Yoga, and why this necessity is the foundation of our resilient nature.

Māyā and the Magic of Our Story

We are made *of* bone and fluid, skin and tissue, organs and electrical impulses, water and air and earth, but what we are made *for* is our story. Our story is what makes us unique; it is our individual enchantment. It is essential that we do the necessary and beautiful work of individuation and, according to Yoga, engage in its "play." The word in Sanskrit is "*lila*," and it is translated as "divine play." There are many ways to unpack the word and its meaning, but suffice it to say, it means that existence is creative, and the act of creating is a very serious, sometimes painful, and always challenging game.

The enchantment is magical, distracting, and easy to forget. The Sanskrit word for this is "*Māyā*," and it means "illusion" or "magic." When the texts of Yoga speak of us existing behind the veil of *Māyā*, the invitation is not to destroy the veil but simply to recognize it. However, we become so enchanted, even enamored by the veil that we forget there is more to our existence. It's important to note that the veil itself isn't bad or wrong. We actually need it. We need the charm of thinking our story is all that there is so that we remain in the game. This paradox is one of the most intriguing and frustrating parts of Yoga. A paradox is an idea that seemingly contradicts itself but is actually true. For example, when we say, "what I know is that I don't know anything," it is at once contradictory and true. The paradox holds space for contradictions to coexist, and as a society, we find it quite unnerving. The idea that we can be both this and that simultaneously goes strongly against one of the most powerful tools in identity's toolbox: that we can only be one thing and not the other. In modern thinking, the prevalent belief is that it is impossible for contradictions to coexist, and to live, we should pick a side and defeat the opposition at all costs rather than "play" in the possibility that all sides exist simultaneously.

It's in this thought process that the *Māyā* of our story becomes an obstacle instead of an enchantment. As we explored in Chapter 3, with the establishment of cognitive bias, we adhere firmly to our stories and eliminate the possibilities of change. We begin to place demands upon our perception to continually align with our narrative and become angry, afraid, or worse when we are challenged to see it differently. Interestingly, this struggle created by *Māyā* is the birthplace of growth and capacity. These instances of which we come to the breaking points of our own tolerance and ideals are the very precipices that we must navigate in order to grow into the recognition of our own illusion. These edges are danger zones, as we are also heavily laden with what the Yogis call *chaya* or shadows. These unclaimed, exiled parts of our story so desperately want to be seen that they sabotage our efforts to recognize them because this would mean that we could then grow beyond them and be free.

Chaya: The Hidden Characters

Psychologically, shadows are akin to the bad angels on our shoulders—always probing us to do the "wrong" thing, to take the unsafe path, to be reckless and even hurtful. You can think of *chaya* as the trolls under the bridge, your own unsavory characters that desire to act out and in defense of your fears, your dissatisfaction, your betrayals, your anger, your pain. At their core, *chaya* are undigested material that has been tossed away or exiled without being given care and attention. They are not evil or bad in essence, but they tend to enact our undeveloped parts that long to be seen and usually go about vying for this attention in ways that affirm our difficulties and dysfunctions. The challenge in working with *chaya* is that in order to assimilate and integrate our shadows, we must first attenuate them. We must be willing to see the parts of ourselves that are unknown even to us and acknowledge their influence and impact on our lives and the lives of those around us.

Chaya by their nature are hidden. They need help to be seen, even though they are always present and often are seen through the observation of others, which feels at times intolerably uncomfortable. They hide from view, even when in plain sight. Working with *chaya* takes patience, diligence, and perseverance to attenuate, assimilate, and integrate them, which will ultimately illuminate these shadows. Often, the most difficult step is witnessing them in action. Turning the light toward and into our dark corners and inky places takes a special kind of courage. We become deep sea divers, daring to submerge into the abyss of our own history, our wounds, our hurts, and our reactivity. We make the choice to meet whatever we find with care and patience and actively resist the judgment and disdain that makes our shadows pull even further away from view.

Little by little, the light of our Yoga begins to shine into the shady spaces, and the *chaya* become more able to sustain the pain of being seen. This is where the process of assimilation can begin. Once we see and acknowledge the shadows within ourselves, we are able to meet them with tenderness, understanding, and acceptance. We no longer wish to exile the hidden bits and instead seek to hear their stories, offer compassion, and space. In doing so, we provide a pathway for the exiled parts of ourselves to return home. Though no less broken and battered by the years of neglect or active disapproval, we allow these concealments to be revealed and meet them with care. This process dismantles the defenses of our shadows and allows recognition and finally ownership to emerge. This is the beginning of integration.

To integrate our *chaya*, we fully own these previously evicted characteristics and allow for our qualities to be fully admitted into the whole of who we are. Rather than continuing to diminish and reduce these aspects within us, we offer space, presence, and eventually agreement. In this way, our shadows are made whole. Creating this wholeness is an act of alchemy that turns our wounds into our weapons (which will be discussed further in Chapters 10 and 11). For now, it is enough to understand that this final step of integration is the experience of Yoga: not the perfected self but the fully integrated one, which is what we experience as resilience. At this point in the process, the *lila* of the universe is embraced. The magic and mystery become the stage for experience rather than things to be feared, and resilience becomes a way of being rather than something to be strived for but never reached.

Lila: The Divine Play of the Universe

An old teaching relayed by one of my earliest teachers says we are put in prison so we may be inspired to find the keys to our own liberation. I am unsure of the origin, but the sentiment appears in many mystical traditions. It reveals the purpose of the struggle (our duty or *dharma*) and points us to the understanding of a much bigger picture than our limited view can perceive. This is the play of the universe, the game of our existence, the unending churn of forgetting and remembering that keeps us engaged and curious, actively pursuing our lives and an understanding of our larger purpose. This is the enchantment of human existence, this is the divine play that calls us not to plot development, things like achievement, success, and perfection, but to the development of our character, our identity, our contribution to the bigger picture.

When attempting to explain *lila* to my students, I use the analogy of an IMAX movie screen. What is real about our existence is what is conveyed onto the IMAX screen, but what we have the capacity to perceive about our existence is a mere pixel on that screen. So, we are always playing a part, always influencing the whole picture, even if only in an infinitesimal way, but part of the play (*lila*) is that we forget. We mistakenly think our pixel is the entire screen, and we live in a way that develops our forgetting. It's important not to directly equate this idea of play with joy or fun. This misconception will create turmoil in trying to understand the nature of the immense tragedies that befall us and those known and unknown to us. Instead, it's more helpful to interpret "play" as a dramatic enactment, such as a play or a movie that engages us in both the bad and the good or an enchantment that requires us to participate.

> What good amid these, O me, O life?
>
> *Answer.*
> That you are here—that life exists and identity,
> That the powerful play goes on, and you may contribute a verse
> ["O Me! O Life!"].
>
> —Walt Whitman

The unique part that we each have to play is called "*svadharma*," "one's own right, duty, or nature; one's own role in the social and cosmic order" (Encyclopedia.com, "Svadharma," n.p.), situated in the *samanya dharma* that deals with the ethical and moral principles of a society and culture (often interpreted as the rule of law), which is, in turn, encapsulated by the "eternal" or absolute set of duties or *sanatana dharma*. One way to think of this is as a map moving from the microcosm out to the macrocosmic understanding of the whole. In other words, it's the characters, the setting, and the set of the play.

When we begin to view the entirety of our experience through this Yogic lens of *dharma* and *lila*, then we begin to transition from the confined cage of individualism into feeling curious about what is beyond the concept of our limited self. This helps us to view our individual identity in terms of communities, cultures, and times that extend beyond us. The result is a buoyancy that allows us to respond to the obstacles and challenges of life through the lens of a bigger picture of both time and place, applying the qualities of rebound and recovery, and to not become so bogged down in the devastation of our individual story. We begin to feel the space that van der Kolk references: "you realize that that something [out there] is not you, so you don't necessarily get hijacked by unpleasant experiences" (Tippett, *Becoming Wise*, p. 88). This is the nature of both resiliency and Yoga.

Practice and Application

Feel and Observe: Take a walk through your neighborhood or town center. Observe how you reference yourself in relationship to your surroundings and the people you encounter. Observe whether you are part of this story or the narrator of it. Consider that you are a piece in the whole of what you are taking in through your eyes, your ears, your nose, and skin. Feel your surroundings as a part of you. Now, feel the impact of *your* contribution to the space through which you are moving. Observe how your presence has subtle influence over the space you occupy.

Inquiry: What role do you play in the bigger picture of your life? What are your contributions to the stories of your family, community, workplace, landscape, and time? What "verse(s)" are you contributing to the "play," even if you don't realize it?

Movement: With music or in silence, stand in the middle of a room, any room. Close your eyes. Beginning with your feet on the ground, begin to feel from the inside out that you are taking up space. From the inside out, begin to expand into the space you occupy. Take up *lots* of space. Begin to move in a way that fills the room you are in: stretch your arms wide, widen your stance, broaden your front and back, maybe even make a sound. If you feel inspired to move in any way (dance, twirl, sing, etc.), follow the inspiration.

Āsana and Energetics Suggestions:
Explore your āsanas *as a way to integrate into the flow of experience* (vyāna).

Chakravākāsana
Bālāsana
Adho Mukha Śhvānāsana
Setu Bandha Sarvāṅgāsana
Matsyāsana
Śhavāsana

58

6

Effort and Ease

The Fallacy of Dichotomy

Resilience requires adaptability to what is and an openness to change, so why are humans so unwilling and averse to change? So many of the ways our model of living is not working have become undeniably apparent in recent years. It is not supporting, adding to, or improving our lives. People pay thousands of dollars in therapy to talk about life, turn it over, understand it, but in the end, many people are, as one of my teachers used to say, more likely to stay in a mediocre level of dysfunction and discomfort than they are to experience the pain of releasing, changing, or growing. So many are afraid of change, not because of what it will bring but because of the sacrifice that will ultimately be required to implement a different way of living. So many are also afraid of taking ownership of the choices they've made that have contributed to their difficulties. Though many are unhappy in their current situation, the discomfort is familiar and, therefore, feels safe and some may even say supportive.

Familiarity gives a sense of comfort based on an innate belief that we can handle what we know. Even when the current situation is unhealthy and painful, so many of us choose to stay enmeshed within those limitations. This refusal to change is often seen as a measure of success and tenacity in our current culture. According to writer Elizabeth Svoboda:

> Most of us have a strong drive to hold on to pre-existing beliefs and convictions, which keep us anchored in the world. When your stance on controversial issues both cements your group identity and plants you in opposition to perceived enemies, changing it can exact a high personal toll ["Why Is It So Hard," n.p.].

We view our positions as fixed, our viewpoints as static, and feel that change is equated with "flip-flopping," "a derogatory term for a sudden real or apparent change of policy or opinion" (Wikipedia, "Flip-flop," n.p.). This fallacy of strength and steadfastness leads to an absence of resilience by limiting our ability to grow from our lessons, to stretch beyond our perceptions, and to be buoyant in times of stress and difficulty and instead leaves us fixed and stuck in positions that we may otherwise have outgrown or surpassed. When our strong convictions become immovable, we are limiting our resilience as well as enforcing one of the obstacles in the experience of Yoga: inflexibility.

One way that resilience is experienced, not taught, is in our ability and willingness to adapt. When something isn't working, we can recall as stated in the previous chapter that resilience is the ability to attenuate (turn toward in order to reduce), assimilate (understand and incorporate), and finally integrate (to form into a new whole) the experience. This is different from dwelling on the problem or strategizing a solution. This is not about "fixing" the brokenness or even healing the wound. In fact, this approach is about honoring the dysfunction, allowing its presence, and changing the way we perceive our problems in order to create a different response. Resilience is about showing up to what is rather than requiring a certain set of conditions to be present before we engage in doing things differently.

This idea of resilience can feel overwhelming when we are firmly fixed to external evidence and reinforcement, and the idea of changing our patterns can seem laborious and destined for failure. The effort required to shift our perspective can seem like "too much work" when weighed against the ease of behaving in the old and familiar ways. Allowing ourselves to consider conflicting ideas and perspectives can bump up against our identity and understanding of "the way things work." It can feel frustrating, aggravating, and even ridiculous, and if we find that our old ways of thinking might be wrong, we experience shame and guilt for not seeing things differently sooner. It seems easier to do things as they've always been done rather than to put effort toward new responses and habits of reaction. It's simpler to do what we've come to know as "right" or avoid what we perceive to be "wrong" than it is to question whether or not these categories of measurement are correct or accurate for our current situation or state of being. After all, most adults have spent the majority of their lives cultivating familiar patterns of response, so it might feel like years or even decades have been wasted if they change their methods, not to mention that there are no guarantees of success. The challenge here is a Yogic one: to understand that no effort or time is ever truly wasted and that every action and inaction, every reaction and response, have contributed to shaping us into the unique people we are now and are essential for our individual stories.

Dynamism Is the Essence

Luckily, resilience isn't measured in categories of opposition or achievement. Resilience isn't based on getting things right or avoiding getting things wrong. Resilience is the willingness to learn from the experience in which we find ourselves without placing requirements on outcome, what the ancient sages of Yoga and other forms of mystical spirituality called "non-attachment" (*Vairāgya*). Being resilient requires risk and allows room for failure, readjustment, education, and learning. Rather than remain in the familiar, resilient people have the courage to try, to take chances, to flunk, to be wrong, and ultimately to change.

The foundation of Yoga (and resilience) is dynamism. The quality or expression of being "dynamic" is "characterized by constant change, activity, or progress" (Lexico, "Dynamic," n.p.). This helps us to understand the idea of Yoga as change rather than as a sense of unchanging steadiness and balance, as it is often explained. The practices of Yoga don't stop change; they embrace it and encourage us to expand our capacity to sustain and thrive in its midst. And this is the very nature of resilience. If we allow our Yoga practices to align us with change and uncertainty, as the dynamic nature of existence directs us to do, then our Yoga will be synonymous with our resiliency. However, when our Yoga becomes the counterpoint to our chaos—the opposite of it rather than the entry point to it—we can find ourselves in a tug-of-war between peace and turmoil, and we are never fully able to inhabit either one due to the pull of the other. Our desires become binary, a one-or the-other situation, a fixed and final position, and, more importantly, they remain infinitely unattainable.

The Resolution of Opposites

This inability to resolve opposites inside and outside reinforces the idea that choosing one or the other is the goal. Yoga teaches us that the point isn't to land on either side of the dichotomy of good or bad, correct or incorrect, right or wrong but to land firmly at the intersection of the either/or conundrum and practice resolving the oppositions. This resolution isn't an immovable destination of one side or the other but is a place where both sides of the opposition are allowed to coexist. When we are able to yoke one side of a position to its opposite, then we are *in* Yoga. From this place, we become buoyant in our choices and decisions, no longer anchored by only one side of an issue or experience.

Yoga of Resilience

This is a challenging viewpoint to comprehend because the invitation is to live within a paradox, live within both sides of a dichotomy at once. The experience of the resolution of opposites opens us up to the discovery of the trust that is available in the mystery of the unknown and, rather than seek security in what we know, to find joy in our sadness or despair in our celebration. When we are aware that every gain contains within it a loss, every success is at once an achievement and a failure, then we are practicing the resolution of opposites. It's a bit like standing in the center of a seesaw and riding the highs and lows of either side while keeping one foot on both sides of the experience. Resolution of opposites requires us to have a relationship with our *chaya* and *Māyā*, to understand that when we are drawn to one side of a thing, it's often an invitation to the other where we find our hidden and forgotten parts that are longing for integration.

This idea of allowing both sides of a belief, opinion, or "truth" to coexist is a radical one, and it is the very heart of Yoga and resilience. Unfortunately, we are not educated to do this until it's almost too late. By the time we begin to unfold this idea, it feels strange and foreign. It is often expressed as a waste of time or energy or as a weakness. The willingness to allow both sides of a thing to be present at once is not a popular opinion in modern culture, but it is the very essence of resilience, and it is the core of Yoga.

Perhaps because it's not efficient or economical to allow resolution as opposed to victory and defeat, our culture teaches us the dangers of failure rather than the lessons of it. We cut our teeth on the endeavor for success and are encouraged to expect nothing less than achievement. We are indoctrinated into a "dog-eat-dog" understanding of the world. These binaries define our existence from the very beginning. But they are showing their impending expiration, as many young people in today's culture are pushing back against this dichotomous worldview. Modern culture has been established within a binary framework in order to secure its investment in itself, primarily in efficient and economical solutions, while it disregards or devalues additional measures of what's possible. Our culture believes that we can perfect our imperfections and, in doing so, attempts to override the fact that you will never be without the challenges of your dysfunctions, failures, or pain. We will never perfect ourselves to such a point that our dysfunctions cease to exist (consciously or subconsciously), and as long as this perfection is the desired result, our dysfunctions (*chaya*) will (and *do*) sabotage our best efforts. If we resist the parts of ourselves that we do not approve of, that we dislike, that are dysfunctional, then resilience is out of our grasp.

62

6. Effort and Ease

It isn't until we can turn toward our resistances that we can truly begin to live in the fullness of possibility, i.e., resilience. When we hold the contradictions of our direct or perceived experience together, in equal measure, without attempting to eliminate one in favor of the other, then we are stepping into the messy and challenging beauty that is Yoga and resilience. There isn't a set group of practices for this, though Yoga provides many exercises that can support the uncomfortable process of assimilating all our parts and moving toward wholeness. Once you are not fighting against yourself, once you are not resisting your pain, sadness, anger, fear, disappointment, then you will be living in a resilient way, you will become more allowing of yourself, and in turn, more allowing of the difficulties of others, and you will model resilience for those who still cling to perfection and resist change at all costs.

I have a friend that refers to this process as "turning into the skid." When an opportunity arises to look your own beliefs and discomforts straight in the eye, you may feel the pain (and sometimes terror) of coming face-to-face with your own unconscious and subconscious beliefs. The risk here is that you will realize your beliefs are "wrong" or just don't fit you anymore. Culturally speaking, the USA is turning into its own in these modern times, with everything from norms of gender orientation, race, and power all coming under review both individually and nationally. The discomfort is almost unbearable at times, but the result is that our culture is changing, shifting, and refining its course. It's repairing (albeit slowly) the damaging beliefs of the past that have been long ignored and making better, more inclusive choices for the future. And, no, this repair is not happening everywhere, it's not happening fast, and it's not happening without resistance, but it is happening, proving that we are capable of expanding our capacity to sit in the discomfort of our own self-reviews and open to the possibility for true and sustainable growth.

This process is achingly slow. For a time in history when all results are expected instantly and perfectly, we struggle to see the micromovements toward change that are blossoming in every moment. Our "skid" is that we demand perfection and that we demand it now or not at all. Somewhere along the way, we were incorrectly taught that to be perfect and to be right were synonymous and that to change our course is an admission of being wrong. So, we learned that rather than adapt (which is a slow and steady process), we must fix what is wrong immediately, choking off the possibility of learning from our mistakes. We have come to believe that rather than change, we must perfect the imperfect thing.

This impulse has led to a deluge of unhelpful behaviors for us and others, such as denying the time necessary to engage in the process of learning (which includes failing), demonizing adaptation, and damning the possibility of true innovation and evolution. As a species, we often feel stuck: caged by our need to be right and for change to be immediate, trapped by our unwillingness to reevaluate what is wrong without being punitive, and kept far away from our resilience even though it is and has always been within us.

Collaboration Instead of Competition

The shift from the primacy of dichotomy into a broader understanding is not as big of a leap as we might think. When we work to apply the tools of attenuation, assimilation, and integration, we cultivate a space where the fullness of experience can be sustained. Be aware that this allowance does not equate to agreement, but it can provide a foundation for understanding, compassion, and empathy even for those with whom we vehemently disagree, even when all our wounds are "triggered," even when we feel unsafe. The resolution of opposites does not disempower our beliefs; instead, it strengthens our conviction. It allows for all things to be considered and our minds to stretch to the edge of our awareness. It builds rather than diminishes; it expands from our collapse.

So where do we begin? Well, with ourselves, of course! We can begin to practice resolving the opposites within us by becoming curious about the things that we resist. In *The Yoga Sūtra of Patañjali*, the author directs us toward several teachings and practices that support this resolution. In sutra 1.33, he encourages the practice of *Pratipakṣha Bhāvanam* or cultivating the opposite feeling.

> *Maitri karuna muditopeksanam sukha duhkha punyapunya visayanam bhavanatas citta prasadanam.*
>
> By cultivating the attitudes of friendliness toward the happy, compassion for the unhappy, delight in the virtuous and disregard toward the wicked, the mind-stuff retains its undisturbed calmness.

Here we are instructed to first bring consciousness to our feelings and responses (attenuation) and then to actively cultivate their opposite. This action allows us not to reduce or diminish our initial reaction but to add to its opposite. Gently we hold both sides together in a way that supports our own expansion.

6. Effort and Ease

In the same text, Patanjali speaks of the five *Kleshas* or causes of affliction. They are:

1. *Avidyā*—often translated as "ignorance" but more precisely interpreted as turning away from or against knowledge or knowing.
2. *Asmitā*—which means our self-identification or attachment to the story of who we are (sometimes mistranslated as "ego").
3. *Raga*—this means attachment to or attraction to our ideas and perceptions of satisfaction (the pursuit of happiness).
4. *Dwesha*—or aversion. This could be thought of as avoidance but could also be looked at through the lens of being attached to what we don't want. *And this is what keeps us attached to our dichotomies so intensely.*
5. *Abhinivesha*—our fear of annihilation. This *klesha* is arguably the origin point for all the rest. In our desperate attempt to avoid our own destruction, we hold tight to what feels good, push away what doesn't, become overly invested in our story (identity), and forget that we are always changing, always inventing, always rewriting the story of our own "truth."

When we dive into the possibility that our aversions are attachments too, we begin to discover how what we avoid also has a hold over us and possibly even a stronger one than that which we desire. We can explore the experience of *dwesha* from an entirely different perspective by looking at our aversions as attachments to what we don't want. It calls on us to look more deeply at our resistances and dislikes and to turn a curious eye toward what we don't want and why. Understanding that we bind ourselves to our resistances helps us to make wiser choices by untangling us from what we avoid and ultimately freeing up space within us to reduce our resistance and open up to new possibilities.

When we are able to recognize that our attachment to certain ideas and our resistance to others doesn't come from a survival place but rather from our attachments, then we unlock the space to be more sensitive to our triggers without pushing them away. Allowing ourselves to feel the responses that we once judged as good or bad, right or wrong, safe or dangerous and move into those feelings rather than identify with them creates the powerful space of acceptance of what is.

Acceptance of what is is the threshold of a resilient life, and it is the experience of Yoga internally.

Practice and Application

Feel and Observe: Be still or make some slow gentle movements or undulations. Feel the right leg. Really give it your attention. Make some movements with it if it helps. Now feel the left leg and all the sensations or vacancies that may be present. Next, feel both legs at the same time. Observe how your mind and perspective must expand in order to feel both legs at once. Stop here or continue on to feel and observe the same process in your arms.

Inquiry: What am I unwilling to change about myself? Why?

Movement: From all fours, move from impulse and inspiration, focusing on the sensations and feelings in your abdomen. Feel your belly rise and fall or circle and shift. Feel its movement in relationship to the floor beneath you. If you move from side to side, can you feel the movement being initiated in your abdomen? If you move backwards and forwards, can you sense this movement emerging from the space behind your naval?

Āsana and Energetics Suggestions:

Explore your āsanas *as a way to renew your vital force and self-awareness* (prāṇa).

Tadāsana
Utkatāsana
Uttānāsana
Prasārita Pādottānāsana
Mālāsana
Adho Mukha Śhvānāsana
Paschimottānāsana
Śhavāsana

7

Truth and Faith

The Misunderstanding of Belief

If acceptance is the gateway to Yoga and resilience, then it might be said that resistance is the barricade. We often resist change and movement in an attempt to create predictability and safety to avoid the unknown. In Yoga as in resilience, it is trust that makes space for us to move, trust that opens us up to undetermined possibility, and trust that generates safety in the experience of risk. We mistakenly equate trust with truth, when, in fact, it might be just the opposite.

Truth and Safety

The attachment to certainty is one of our primary obstacles to resilience and to the experience of Yoga. In our quest for creating stability, we often bypass the experience of uncertainty that can guide us to deepening levels of understanding, learning, and freedom. Because complexity often feels overwhelming, we strive to distill the intricate down to simple and manageable truths that cannot be argued against in order to feel safe and secure on the bedrock of our beliefs. Unfortunately, the belief systems that give us such a strong sense of safety are the very same understandings that trap us in cycles of fear, control, and demand. The systems that are meant to be the foundation on which we stand and grow become the quicksand that pulls us away from the vast spectrum of what's possible.

The gap between what is "true" and what is "real" is an enigmatic one that Yoga directs us to question constantly. Recognition of the diversity of perspectives intertwining and engaging is what creates the richness of our aliveness. In an effort to establish a single truth, system, or belief, we rob ourselves of the immensity of experience and ultimately the capacity to grow and learn. Adherence to a specific understanding (or truth) as absolute is the basis of a belief system that is not contraindicated in Yoga, and in some cases it's even necessary. But, when our belief systems become rigid and fixed, when they become ways to ensure safety, when we demand beliefs to be unchanging and truth to be fixed, we are engaging in the very thing that Yoga advises us against: an ignorance (*Avidyā*) of the ever-changing and complex nature of existence. Resilience makes space for this sort of complexity and allows for the diversity of belief systems to coexist without the requirement of agreement. Interestingly, it's this very diversity and disagreement that open the doors to faith. Allowing this complexity teaches us to trust and discern from our inner truth, to calibrate our compass inward, to shelter our beliefs deep within, to truly feel them rather than performing rote action, and ultimately to align our actions in harmony with both our hearts and our world.

Interpretations of Faith

Yoga describes faith as *sraddha*, meaning specifically trust in those who have walked the path before you. That faith is an active rather than passive response to the absence of certainty and can be based in systems of belief and learning, as well as direct observation and experimentation.

In our modern culture, faith is often expressed as blind adherence to a set of rules or systems, a relinquishing of agency. When we understand faith in this way, we seek an external force to save us from our pain or travail. We embrace our beliefs as authoritative, actively ignoring our doubt or discernment, and we hand over our autonomy. At the extreme end of the spectrum, we may even perceive ourselves as powerless to engage. This understanding of faith often results in a conflict wherein we are fully dependent upon systems outside of us to improve our situation as well as victimized by their inability or unwillingness to help or change our predicament. Faith of this kind paradoxically strengthens the belief in the systems of salvation and weakens the trust and agency of the individual. It's a cycle, as so many things are, that keeps us chasing the unattainable when we should slow down and dare to inquire about the efficacy or support in that which we place our faith.

The recognition that reality may be bigger than we think or perceive (or have been taught) leads to all sorts of mental tugs-of-war between what we believe and what is "true." These mental acrobatics can shake the core of belief even for those who feel firm in their foundation and elicit an awareness that our understandings are not infallible nor are they ever truly complete. This "crisis of faith" is a necessary process in the maturation of our understanding and belief and is the initiation into an expanded or revised belief system.

When faith is used to avoid the crisis of its own making, it can create rigidity of belief and an inherent mistrust in self-knowledge and inner guidance. It becomes a passive and complacent stance rather than an active and dynamic investigation. It abandons agency and puts the demands of correction upon that which is beyond oneself. This creates a false sense of safety as it waives all self-responsibility or accountability in the given situation thus preventing the faithful from having any culpability for the situation in which they find themselves. The idea that with faith we can do no wrong becomes the predominant sentiment that validates inaction and subverts responsibility, maintaining a perpetual state of oppression for which blame can only be placed outside of us.

Truth then becomes one thing rather than a multifaceted expression of countless perspectives weaving together to create a unique and alive reality. Our limits begin to dictate our experiences rather than the other way around, and we find ourselves trapped in the safety of our cage. We are never really secure and never truly free. This is the opposite of resilience, and it is the entrapment that Yoga seeks to liberate us from. Yoga asks us to acknowledge our systems of belief and simultaneously dares us to question them. It drives us to yoke our certainty to our uncertainty, to unify our doubt with our belief, not in an effort to wipe one or the other away but with the intention of building the capacity for coexistence. Yoga says we do not have to eliminate one side of the experience to fully engage with and inhabit the other. It guides us not to simply walk the path of those that came before but to inquire, to become curious, to adapt, to evolve, and to take the reins of our choices by establishing informed trust.

There is a popular cartoon that illustrates this predicament. A man is drowning in the ocean, desperately praying to God to be saved. A few moments later a life raft paddles by and asks the drowning man whether they can help. The man replies, "No. God will save me." The man continues to struggle, calling louder for God to save him. An ocean liner passes by with a crewmember shouting, "Sir, can we help?" to which the man replies, "No! God will save me." As the man weakens in his struggle, he floats by an island, all the while continuing to call out to God to save him. Predictably, the next scene is of the man, standing at the so-called "pearly gates" and explaining to the gatekeeper how he ended up in heaven. "I prayed for God to save me," he says, "but, alas, He didn't." The gatekeeper laughs and says, "What are you talking about?! God came as a life raft, an ocean liner, and an island." Sometimes we become so focused on the precise outcome we hope to achieve that we forget that we are receiving the opportunities every step of the way.

Faith and Surrender

The teaching on surrender is one of the most misunderstood and misinterpreted teachings in Yoga and in many great mystical traditions. Patanjali references surrender in the last of the five *niyamas,* the second limb of the eight-limbed path of Yoga, when he offers the teaching on Ishvara Praṇidhāna. The word "ishwara" is translated as a generalized term for divinity, akin to the English word "Lord," and *"praṇidhāna"* means to "lay on, fix, apply, attention (paid to), meditate upon, desire, or pray." What is often interpreted as surrender is the action of applying attention to or meditating upon a force that is bigger than us. This encapsulates the Yogic idea of surrender, which is not to give up or even to let go but rather to actively remember (*Smaraṇa*) that we are a part of something much bigger. And as a spoke to a wheel, our function is essential. This bigger force is not only an influencer but also influenced by our active engagement with it. Therefore, surrender is an active process of engagement with that which is bigger than us. It's a verb. Surrender is the action of surrendering rather than a noun or object of achievement. It's remembering that no matter how big our stories seem (and rightfully so sometimes), they are still only a sentence in a much bigger story.

This idea of surrender inevitably leads us back to "truth," the deep and innate knowing that resonates inside us and speaks to us within the context of each and every situation. From truth, we can find the ground of trust that will allow us to continually and perpetually inquire into the validity of our feelings, reactions, and responses. Surrender is a freedom rather than a sacrifice. This is the surrender that Yoga points us to and that resilience provides us the lived experience of. It's not an acquiescence but an activation, a recognition, a remembrance, and it empowers us to embark upon actions that might seem radical in the systems of belief with which we engage. It questions but not necessarily answers, and it allows for the vacancy of answers, which increases our curiosity and our awareness.

Surrender, trust, and truth are gateways to humility, not to be confused with weakness. The tools applied when we surrender are courage, vulnerability, honesty, and willingness: the very tools that pose the greatest risk to belief systems that are shored up with demands for compliance and fidelity. When we are able to understand the depth of power that trust and faith give us access to, as us, from us, and for us, then we are no longer required to diminish ourselves to show our faith. In fact, when we truly begin to discover our essence, we are the emanation of liberation, not because we have transcended anything but because we have landed squarely in ourselves.

Reconciling Belief Brings Us to Reality

When we are able to return to ourselves as the source of our knowing, there is room for all belief systems to thrive. We can dare to question the things we know or have been taught and arrive at our own conclusions that aren't based on what we "should" do or what we are "supposed to" do. We can access inner resources when the ground of our belief becomes shaky and stay open to learning more as we grow beyond the confines of allegiance and loyalty. In this reconciliation, there is room for expansion and inclusion without compromising what is true for us. There is more space for others' belief systems to coexist in harmony with our own. There is a willingness and perhaps even a commitment to the multifarious expressions of belief, truth, and faith, none of which require a singular way to be dominant.

Shifting in this way is challenging but not impossible. It does not require agreement, only willingness to listen and see the many paths of "truth." A good example of these many paths is maybe one of the most difficult to listen to: family. But when we learn to listen and to hear our family members who vocalize wildly different opinions and views than our own without requiring them to change their minds, without withdrawing our love and care, without denying or diminishing our own beliefs, and without shutting down the possibility of changing our own minds, we are in the process of reconciliation. This skillset, though incredibly challenging to cultivate, allows all sides of reality to be included and makes space for what's possible. The more emotionally charged the subject, the more difficult it is, and of course, we all succeed sometimes and fail other times. The success of reconciliation is in the power of the return. If we allow charged disagreements to push us away from our loved ones, we should do the work necessary to return. We should contemplate all sides and check our own indignation. Then we can come back to the table with understanding and perhaps even an expanded view of the conversation.

In resolving our misunderstandings about belief, we come to

appreciate the differences in our views. This is the recognition that Yoga guides us to: that which is bigger (macrocosm) expresses itself as the particular and unique beauty of the individual instance (microcosm). We no longer have to cleave to our individual belief systems for protection and can instead feel safe to inquire, to be curious, and even to change. We no longer risk losing what is real and true as a result of outside influence because we are anchored in a knowing that comes from within.

When belief enhances our lived experience rather than protects us from it, we are able to move with grace and ease in what is real. The real is the unchanging and actual expression of any situation. It is what happens aside from the entrapments of interpretation or analysis. The real just is. It's not changeable based on belief or denial. The rain makes things wet. That's real. The flowers bloom to propagate their species. That's real. And these real expressions and situations are the basis of every experience onto which we apply our personal and individual perspective and belief systems. When we reconcile our beliefs within ourselves, when we dare to wrestle with the questions of doubt and choose to be curious, then we are choosing to live in and with what is real and to carry with us our personal interpretations without the demand that they are the only ones. Living in what is real is what Yoga teaches us. We don't have to like it, but we can't escape it. Reference points calibrated toward the deep internal center allow us to live even in the harshest of realities, even amidst pain and heartbreak, even when we feel oppressed. Living in this way is resilience. It is Yoga.

Practice and Application

Feel and Observe: Call to mind a disagreement. Observe how your body responds to even the thought of a difference of opinion. Feel what tightens, feel how your breath changes, feel how your pulse responds. Observe these feelings as *yours* in response to a recollected experience and become aware of how you respond to the feelings rather than the information that initiated it.

Inquiry: Which of your beliefs are truly yours? How do you know? How do you respond when your beliefs are challenged? Where did you learn to do that?

Movement: Cover your eyes with a scarf, eye mask, or blindfold. Bring yourself to sit, stand, or lie down in a space that's clear of obstacles. Once more become aware of the feelings that arise from inside your body when your beliefs are challenged. Now, without referencing your external environment, move into the felt sensations of challenge in your body. Allow your movement to be a response to what you are feeling inside. If thoughts surface, trace them to their expression in your body, then allow yourself to move into and with those expressions. The movements could be small or imperceptible or they could be big or even loud. Whatever they are, keep checking that they are initiated from inside rather than directed from outside of you.

Āsana and Energetics Suggestions:

Explore your āsanas as a way to assimilate and integrate from the inside out (samāna/vyāna).

Try these suggestions blindfolded

Chakravākāsana
Bālāsana
Baddha Koṇāsana
Upaviṣṭa Koṇasana
Adho Mukha Śhvānāsana
Sphinx
Jaṭhara Parivartanāsana
Legs Up the Wall
Śhavāsana

8

The Tool of Hope

When belief and faith are needed, hope is often where we turn to save us from our challenges or difficulties. In today's lexicon, hope is often interpreted as positivity or optimism, synonymous with a "wish," but is rarely employed as a tool to engage with directly. Hope as a tool has a different purpose and pursuit. When applied to the practices of the recognition of what is real and the reconciliation of belief, hope is an instrument of trust. Contrary to the interpretation of hope in terms of a positive outcome or wish fulfillment, hope is a space that is free of requirements. At its heights, it allows for alignment with our center without losing the awareness of what is. It does not demand or expect, and it does not require specific outcomes in order to be employed. The tool of hope arrives wherever we are and holds space for what is possible. It is relentless in its commitment to the unseen and enigmatic, and it's committed to possibility beyond proof. Hope as a tool is not a dream or fantasy; it's the crack or fissure in all experiences where potential is available beyond what is perceived.

When hope enters into the resilience equation, it stretches beyond the known patterns of behavior and into the application of lessons learned and opportunities to explore faith rather than reduce a given obstacle to a puzzle of logic or victimhood. Hope is best utilized as a method to expand what's available to be known rather than an attempt to remedy what is not known. Hope can be a bridge into the frightening and unfamiliar territory of the unknown, lightening the weight of the loads that we carry and widening our sights. However, hope is not dependent upon a positive outcome. When used appropriately, hope is untethered to result and invites into more.

For so many, "hope is a thing with wings." It's the thing that "floats" above the fray. In the modern world of overwhelming determinism, hope has become a way to escape the sometimes unbearable pain of what's real and to bypass our agency and responsibility. We often "hope" that things will work out in lieu of working with the discomfort that's right in front of us. We send our hopes toward others when we feel helpless and wait to see if they return to us in ways that will lead us to fulfillment. Hope as an expectation or goal can leave us feeling disappointed and dejected when our plan doesn't work out, but hope as a tool can be utilized with different effects.

When we begin to understand that hope isn't an antonym of loss or grief but rather the point of connection to our desire, then we find power in our hope rather than helplessness, as we will explore in the following chapter. Hope can become an entry point into the difficulty of pain and suffering, a flashlight that illuminates a way when we are groping in the darkness. When hope is utilized as a tool, it resists its affiliation to salvation and compels us instead to become active participants in that for which we hope.

The Relationship of Hope and Surrender

Surrender, as discussed in the previous chapter, is a word that—though referenced often in modern Yoga—is rarely, if ever, understood, and even rarer still is surrender actually experienced. As one of my teachers told me almost two decades ago, surrender cannot be taught; it can only be experienced directly. Yet, time and time again, in Yoga classes and beyond, we are given the instruction to "let go," often with the added diminishment of the phrase "just" as in "just let go," as if this is the easiest and simplest thing we could do. When expressed as a directive without any further instruction or information, this is a clear cue that the person giving such guidance has never truly experienced surrender for themselves. Surrender, I will boldly declare at the risk of negative feedback, is *not* the same as letting go. Not. Even. Close.

Though surrender may be a release, it's not always a relief. It is a way of entering, not a leaving behind. It's impactful but often quickly forgotten, as true surrender flies in the face of a culture based on lack, fear, salvation, and achievement. Surrender is not a letting go but a letting be. It's not a release as much as an arrival. It sets free only that which never really was and provides the space and permission to participate with reality. True surrender does not discharge your debts and obstacles; it gathers them up, harnesses them into a space of reclamation in order to be met fully and collaborated with as a means to move onward as who we really are. Surrender requires a petition for truth, an agreement that we will allow and acknowledge the full scope of reality in which we find ourselves. Surrender admits our faults and failures, it concedes to our defeats and downfalls, and it grants permission for the truth of a situation to exist. It does not wish it away or pray for change. It does not let go but rather holds fast to the fullness of the story. It does not release the burden of the truth but rather willingly shoulders the weight of reality as a recognition that where we are is much bigger than we can comprehend.

The tool of hope best serves surrender as the way to engage with that which is beyond what we know about ourselves and others. Hope calls us into the space that is bigger than our small dramas and into the grand arena of the possible. Hope works with surrender by allowing us to see more in ourselves than reality makes apparent and by opening us up to the possibility that we are more than we thought. In turn, surrender helps us to similarly recognize this bigger role for others, regardless of evidence to the contrary. Hope as a tool is ferocious. It does not back down in the face of contempt or contention. It growls, it howls, and it rises not above the rubble but from within it.

What Hope Is

Hope as a tool is a powerful expression of resilience. Hope commits to more than what can be seen. It conspires with the mystery of which we are a part but can never fully know. Hope is the willingness to dance (*lila*) across the tightrope of danger and to imagine beyond the threat in order to allow the truth of what *is* to cohabitate with the unseen potential of the unknown—the perpetually mysterious, thriving, writhing creative existence of which we are undeniably a part. Hope is the conjunction that joins surrender to trust. And from it, we find our desires that rumble deep within us become clearer and clearer and that they are not dependent upon or diminished by our environment, our safety, or our achievements.

The tool of hope emerges from the fundament of surrender as an active and alive choice. It doesn't wait for the external world to provide for its existence but is evidenced in the action of hoping. The act and expression of hoping, when done well, is defiant. It refutes logic and evidence, it is bigger than what is measurable, and it refuses to fear its own failure. In this way, the tool of hope is a powerful teacher reminding us that the act alone is enough and that it does not require success to be valued or worth the effort.

What Hope Is Not

Our modern, colonized world has a different approach to hope. And I am just a small contributor to the thoughts on the subject. Revered Buddhist nun, Pema Chodron, actually advocates against hope. In her book, *When Things Fall Apart*, she expresses the idea of hope as an obstacle to being where or who we truly are. She proposes that real wisdom begins with hopelessness, and she has a point. Her notion of hope as an impediment to true knowing encapsulates the idea that hope is resignation rather than a tool for action, which emerges from the finality of surrender.

Hope, when used as a tool of engagement, is not an object or even a subject. In fact, it's not a thing at all. Hope as a tool is an action, which emerges from the rocky bottomed pit of self-knowing. Hope is a "doing" that meets "being" right where it is and does not require change to exist. It's the recognition that there is always more than we know, and it's the invitation to the active engagement with what is beyond our small self-story. Hope, in this context, is not wishful thinking. It does not dig in its heels and wait for a savior. It does not deny the truth of what is; it simply expands it into the spaces that our small minds and limited perspectives cannot comprehend.

Hope as a tool is diligent and steadfast. It shows up in the darkest of places and reminds us that the light does not cease to exist simply because we cannot see it. Rather than hope being that which parts the clouds of our doubt and despair, hope may be the clouds themselves, an invitation to remember that there is more beyond that which obscures our vision and to remain committed to it regardless of the torrent that is unleashed. Hope tracks the movements of days, seasons, births and deaths, beginnings and endings. Hope is not the antidote to despair; it's the collaborator. Hope is remembering that even when we are in the depths of our sorrows, the story is bigger than us. Hope is the bridge across the abyss, equally committed to both despair and elation, creating the tension needed to keep us moving within the ever-expanding experience of the present-moment reality. It's the music to which we can dance rather than the silence in which to rest.

Working with Hope

Embarking on a practice of hope might seem artificial and contrary if we are committed to a worldview of victimization and power dominance. In many ways, hopelessness might feel like the safer choice, one which is guaranteed not to disappoint. While that may be true, the path of resilience compels us to eschew safety as the goal and take the risk of stepping into the truth of what is without the necessity of security and often without our familiar patterns of protection.

> Start close in ...
> the step you don't want to take
> [*River Flow*].
> —David Whyte

As with most suggestions in this book, working with hope can begin simply, small, and "close in." We all have those edges of despair that nibble at our toes and tug at our hearts. We all have the unspoken fears that preoccupy the silence and creep into the moments of light and inspiration. Maybe it's doubt or failure or pain or suffering, but we all have spaces within us where the tool of hope could be put to use. At first, we may not be skillful, and mistakes will be inevitable, but over time, hope as a tool will become familiar. With practice and diligence, hope as an object to be made manifest will be replaced with hope as an action of holding space for a bigger reality that we can't see. This action does not require our troubles or our fears to disappear but instead includes them as a piece of a bigger possibility.

When we allow the wound, which hides in the shadows and is threatened by change, to step out of its protective covering into the light of the unknown, slowly it begins to recover. This is what the tool of hope offers. Not an absence of the pain or fear that plagues but an inclusion and integration of it that opens space for more. This is resilience: the refusal to hide away from the life that we cannot see or know, the willingness to resist the automatic reactions of protection or control, to take the chance to be hurt again and again, and to meet that pain with hope every time.

To engage with our lives resiliently, the tool of hope is one of the sharpest in our toolbox. Though it does not placate or soothe, it will bolster our efforts. When the world seems hopeless, we bear down with hope to create an opening for more. When we feel bound and stuck in our situation, hope is the end of the fiber that we can tug to unravel the knot. Hope is most helpful when it is least possible, and it is most potent when it supports us as we enter into a given situation head on and heart forward.

The Importance of Energy

The tool of hope can be understood as a type of energy. It is a felt sense of the possible, and it expands what is available, even in the moments when our world seems irrefutably shrunken and tight. "Energy," by definition, is "power derived from the utilization of … resources" and "the strength and vitality required for sustained … activity" (Lexico, "Energy," n.p.). Hope can be both resource and vigor, and as it is energy, it is generative. When you invite hope into hopeless situations, you initiate the opportunity to shift not the situation but your relationship with it.

When you feel stuck in a situation that offers you no easy way out, hope allows you to change your view. Conceding that perhaps we don't have all the answers to our troubles and daring to wonder about them provides an opportunity to see our predicaments in different ways. This tiny opening can free our deadlocked system to receive the tiniest pinprick of possibility and shift our perspective completely. Here is an example: When I have lost something, like my keys, I try and try to think of where I left them. I search and become increasingly irritated at myself and pressured by the situation that caused me to need them in the first place. Sooner or later, I am stuck and feeling hopeless. I acquiesce to the reality that no amount of strategy or effort to solve the problem loosens its grip. But if I sit down, quiet my mind, deepen my breath, and remove the focus from the debacle of my lost keys for even a few moments and allow myself to feel hopeful that I will eventually find them, I am often surprised by the impulse of recollection that points me in the needed direction (and often to a place that I had never even considered).

The energy you bring to any relationship is impactful and generative. If you concede to hopelessness, the energy contained within that choice supports the impact and generation of hopelessness, giving it inertia and inevitably deepening feelings of despair and stagnation and all the other ways hopelessness expresses itself. But when you invite hope in, you invite the paradoxical possibility that more is available than you can see. I reiterate: it doesn't change your circumstances, but it can change your relationship with them and put you back into the driver's seat of your choices.

That tiny shift of perspective is enough to change the way you engage with the dynamic of a situation. This shift is an energetic one and does not occur in the elusive and esoteric way that you might think. Shifting energy means opening your receptors to resources and power. It's a plant sending roots down into the darkness of the soil as well as shoots and leaves up to the warmth of the sun. Energy is felt in a myriad of ways. Expressed through the lens of emotion, it is colored by past interpretations and experiences and then overlaid onto the present. Energy is felt, both inside and out. It is the foundation of action (any action, from running to pushing a baby stroller to typing on a keyboard to launching a rocket), and it is the impulse that precedes thought and feeling. Energy as electricity fires between synapses in the brain (as well as other physical locations) to send and receive messages, to communicate on multiple levels. Energy is like breathing: it's both automatic (unconscious) and can be controlled by attention and action (conscious). This is why energy is equated with breath in Yoga. Prāṇa (meaning "energy" in Sanskrit) is often reduced to the breath in description and definition, but it is much more than that: it is every vibrating atom of existence. It is you and me and the top of the mountain. Amazingly overlooked, it is the fullest potential of every moment, and when we choose to bring our unconscious into our conscious awareness, we have access to it and a choice about how we use it.

The tool of hope holds within it the possibility of change, though it is impossible to control or define. When refined and sharpened, the tool of hope offers the possibility of a widening perspective that creates space to make choices, reflect, engage, and even evolve. What is necessary for hope to be a tool rather than a wish or escape, however, is an approach that is free from expectation of outcome.

Yoga Is Energy Management

Yoga is a system of energy management. It is a method of practice and living that puts our engagement with energy at the forefront of our experiences and asks us to bring consciousness to the ways we shape, move, refine, and express it. It provides tools to respond from the full scope of our energetic experiences rather than reduce our intelligence to just the mental, physical, or emotional. The energy to which I refer is not an esoteric or New Age concept. The energy of Yoga refers to the very same energy that composes the building blocks of all things—what the Greek philosophers first identified and named "atoms."

The energy of Yoga follows all the same rules and laws as the energy of science because it is the same. We are made up of these building blocks, just as the rocks and oceans and even the air are. We are unceasingly vibrating, resonating, and moving with and as energy and so is everything and everyone around us. When we are able to engage and respond from this level of awareness, we shift from being merely thinking beings with bodies into beings of full-bodied intelligence. We awaken the capacity of the entirety of ourselves to "know" and "learn." We become more sensitive to the experiences in which we find ourselves, and through the practice of Yoga, we act in, from, and with this place consciously.

8. The Tool of Hope

The practice of energy management in Yoga is called "prāṇāyāma," meaning control or restraint of the life-force energy. Though usually equated with breathing techniques, the practice of prāṇāyāma is a much larger invitation to bring consciousness to the full scope of our interactions, both within and outside of us. Working with prāṇa gains us access to the "more" that Yoga tells us is accessible in all things at any time. It expands our understanding to that which can be perceived as energy in any given context, and it empowers us to respond in equal measure. When we have a basic understanding of Yogic energetics, we are able to engage with and from this understanding in a way that generates a significant impact.

The Yogis had complex and specific ways of understanding *prāṇa*, its movement and its influence, and its relationship to our physical, mental, and emotional systems. Yoga's sister science, *Ayurveda*, states that humans are made up of a combination of three primary constitutions or *doshas* (which literally translates as "defects"): *Vāta*, *Pitta*, and *Kapha*. Our unique combination of these three foundational expressions is what makes us who we are. The depth of *Āyurveda* is immense, and its scope well exceeds what I can cover here. But in an attempt to summarize a very complex system of health, lifestyle, and body practices, a brief explanation of the *doshas* is as follows: *Vāta* is a combination of the elemental energies of air and space, *Pitta* combines the elemental energies of water and fire, and *Kapha* is the combined qualities of earth and water.

The Yogic approach of energetics looks primarily through the lens of *Vāta Doṣha* with prāṇa being expressed in five distinct ways called the "*prāṇa vāyus*" ("prāṇa," meaning "energy"; "*vāyu*," meaning "wind"). The *prāṇa vāyus* tell us a great deal about our internal relationships with energy and help us to derive more clarity about how to engage with that energy. I will provide more in-depth explanations of the *prāṇa vāyus*, their functions, and how to work with them in Chapter 15. For now, it's helpful to understand our capacity to release, sustain, and build energy as an essential component of our relationship with hope, and awareness of the energy to which we have access or from which we feel estranged is directly related to our potential to envision more.

When our energy is stagnant or "low" (meaning we have low access to our available energy), we often express this inertia as hopelessness, despair, sadness, and depression. We find it next to impossible to apply the tool of hope and can feel powerless to change the experiences, situations, and perceptions in which we find ourselves. This condition is colloquially described as "not seeing the forest for the trees." We become so bound in our current state of experience and its relationship to our past difficulties that we struggle to pull our head above the details of what we can perceive directly and access the potential that lies beyond that. An understanding of the *vāyus* helps us identify where, why, and how our energy is impacting our experience and expression, and it empowers us make conscious alterations. All the practice suggestions in this book have worked with and will continue to work with your energy through the lens of the *prāṇa vāyus* to help provide the tools for you to hone in on the subtle but powerful forces within and utilize them effectively.

The tool of hope is the doorway to this potential, and understanding how to use and shift our relationship with energy can be the key that turns the lock. Yoga offers us instructions, guides, anecdotes, mythologies, and space to build our capacity to see beyond the limitations of our perceptions and to open up to more than what we previously recognized as possible. Opening, receiving, and allowing for more makes us resilient yet realistic. We don't have to be overly optimistic or positive to create space for each moment to hold more than we can recognize; we simply have to be available for a truth beyond our perception or control. Hope grants us access to the mysterious without the safety net of guarantees. It holds the door open without forcing us to cross the threshold. It encourages us to lift our eyes to see what is beyond our singular perception of any given situation and allows us to see ourselves as a part of something bigger without having to know what that is.

Practice and Application

Feel and Observe: Feel the sensation of your breath rising and falling through your nostrils. Feel the inhale pass over the tips of the nostrils and rise through the nasal passages, and now feel the exhale leave through the nasal passages and pass again over the tips of the nostrils. Observe the breath in this way for a few moments. Now, sense that the nostril is a cylinder, and feel the breath passing over the ceiling of the cylinder. Refine your awareness to feel the subtle experience of the breath passing over the ceiling of the cylinder of the nasal passage. Observe how this refined awareness extends beyond the gross sensation of the breath and accesses something more subtle but no less present.

Inquiry: Where in your life do you feel hopeless? Where do you desire more hope? How can you utilize the tool of hope to discover new possibilities?

8. The Tool of Hope

Movement: Lie on your back on the floor and squeeze your knees into your abdomen, holding them in with your hands. Feel yourself bound up tight, unable to move. Now, without force, begin to feel the spaces that exist even within the squeeze (at the crease behind the knees, at the flexing hips, at the ankles, or in the back of the body). Then, begin to expand and move your breath into the spaces that you discovered, allowing the places to ever so slightly expand with each inhale. Allow the spaces to grow with each consecutive breath until they feel stronger and more powerful than the grip against them. Release your hands and allow the legs to release and move as they desire. Follow that movement through your whole body.

Āsana and Energetics Suggestions:

Explore these āsanas *as a way to build enthusiasm and hopeful expression* (udāna).

Chakravākāsana
Tadāsana
Trikonāsana
Śhalabhāsana
Sphinx
Setu Bandha Sarvāṅgāsana
Matsyāsana
CRP

Want, Desire, and Longing
Are Not the Same Thing

Reading the Messages of Emotion

We live in a culture of insatiable want. We want it all, we want it bigger and better, we want it now. The word "want" appears in seven out of the 10 most recent news headlines appearing on Google as I write this, referring both to achievement and loss. We feel that we deserve to have what we want, and we work tirelessly to get it. We value our freedom to want more for ourselves and our children. We identify with our wants and validate them with our words and actions. To want is the American way, and it might be one of the most significant hurdles of resilience.

From a Yogic perspective, words hold power. Sounds and syllables create vibrations that attract, repel, and resonate. The language of Yoga is Sanskrit, and each letter of the alphabet has a specific vibration and resonance. Alone and in combination, they contain the power and meaning of the entire universe. Though the English language isn't viewed through the same sacred lens, the idea that our words have impact can be evidenced in all the great spiritual philosophies and beyond. Because of the power of words, it's worthwhile in this exploration of the Yoga of resilience to be curious about the language of resilience and to investigate how bringing awareness to even the simplest things has a great impact.

Want Versus Desire

The word "want" comes from the Old Norse root *vantr*, meaning "to lack." When we advocate for what we want, we are pleading our lack of it. Wanting expresses absence and reinforces the vacancy by demand. When we feel the pull of wanting, we are being invited to investigate our relationship with scarcity. Is what we seek really going to be sufficient to fulfill our perceived deficit? Or do we need to do the work of inquiring more deeply, attenuating our attractions, assimilating our lack, and integrating our understanding into the whole? If we discover that we do not actually lack what we want, then our want might unfold into something more akin to desire. "You are what your deepest driving desire is. As your desire is, so is your will. As your will is, so is your deed. As your deed is, so is your destiny" (*Brihadaranyaka Upanishad* 4.4).

Yoga has many teachings on desire, from overcoming it to succumbing to it; the notion is pervasive in the texts. So, what is desire, really? "Desire" comes from the Latin roots *de*, meaning "down," and *sitare*, meaning "stars." The experience of desire in Yoga is directly related to the expression of dharma, which we discussed in Chapter 5. Desire is a pull toward purpose. Both the individuated purpose and the universal one are served when we become aware and engaged with our desire. Desire doesn't emerge from absence but is an expansion or enhancement of the recognition of our role in the whole. We desire what will bring us into greater alignment with who we truly are. We desire what will engage us in a deeper way with what is and what will bring us more into concert with our expression. It is the path of our unique reflection of place and action when it is made manifest within the bigger context. To recognize and honor our desires is a type of service to the whole, a resonance with the bigger picture. As we decrease the dissonance between expression and our desire, the benefit extends well beyond the individual.

Desire Versus Longing

Desire is the song of our individuated soul, according to the *Brihadāraṇyaka Upaniṣad*, but it is distinct from that within us that is bigger than our individuation. The pull to what is beyond us is experienced not as desire but as longing. Mystical teachings tell us that longing is the direct experience of our relationship with something bigger: call it "God," call it "spirit," call it the "great mystery." When we are immersed in longing, we are having an experience of that for which we long. Longing is how we engage with a world that is bigger than our personal experience.

"Longing" comes from the Old English *langian*, meaning "grow long, prolong" and also "dwell in thought, yearn" (Lexico, "Long," n.p.). It has Germanic origin in the word "*langen*," related to the same term in Dutch, which means "reach or extend" and "to present or offer," respectively. To long for something is to dwell in the thought of it, to make an offering, to surrender into the thing for which we long. To long for something is to be in a relationship with it. Whyte says this: "Longing is nothing without its dangerous edge..." (*Consolations*, p. 104).

From the perspective of Yoga, longing is the primal power that fuels life. It is ours to access always and is only as far away as our awareness of it. It is not something to satiate but something to enter, to turn toward as a resource rather than an affliction to cure, and it is the remedy for our over-extension, our separation, our exhaustion, and our loneliness. It seems paradoxical, of course, that we would turn toward longing to find our belonging, but it is precisely this observance that calls us to leave behind our attachment to outcome, identity, and safety in order to move with greatest ease in the world. The prefix "be-" amplifies its root word. It intensifies whatever the root word is expressing. To belong, we intensify our relationship with that for which we yearn. We become intimate with the pull toward the experience, the person, the place, and we strive to be present with it until understanding unfolds.

Longing and Resilience

As Whyte's words express, longing is a risky thing. To enter into a relationship with your longing is perilous. And it requires courage because this relationship leads to encounters with the unknown and mysterious realizations that will emerge. This is the essence of resiliency: to not have it all figured out, healed, or perfected and to nonetheless engage with the pain of our history and to choose, over and over again, to return to the magnetic force of our own hunger. To turn toward our difficulties rather than away from them is to ultimately understand that all these troubles are the source of our power.

Yoga says that desire can open the door to our longing. We can follow who we truly are at our deepest levels and discover what our soul calls for so that we can cultivate a relationship with that calling. It's a path fraught with discomfort and freedom. It's a place where we are fully engaged with all the complex aspects of our experience without losing ourselves. It's overflowing with sensation and feeling, and the only way to truly know our longings is to dare to feel into them.

Because our modern Western culture is cautious towards and distrustful of feeling, this requirement to anchor our feelings toward our longings is where the peril emerges. In my own experience, there is often an association of emotional expression with weakness and a misunderstanding that vulnerability is akin to frailty. We have been taught to have a "stiff upper lip" and that it's a bad thing to wear "our hearts on our sleeves." Perhaps because our modern culture lacks the resources and skills to deal with emotion as it arises, we choose instead to pack it away, to refuse it when it comes, and to numb it until it is beyond recognition. Feelings have come to be defined as unstable and untrustworthy to the point that many people struggle to even identify their own. Many of the students I work with express a strikingly similar difficulty in the realm of feeling, which is expressed in the simple question, "How do I know if I can trust what I'm feeling?" It's an amazing question to which we can apply the distinctions of want, desire, and longing. When was the last time you were conscious of this distinction in your daily life? Try this: the next time you express a want, ask yourself, "Is it true that I lack this?" If the answer is yes, try asking, "Why do I want it?" Sometimes this simple inquiry can help to untangle us from the misunderstandings of want and desire and even direct us to our longing.

Patanjali speaks of this torment as an affliction or *klesha*, which we explored in Chapter 6 along with the five primary causes of affliction: *Avidyā* or ignorance of the truth of our existence; *Asmita*, which is comparable to our general understanding of ego or self-identification; *raga*, meaning attachment; *dwesha*, aversion; and *Abhinivesha*, the fear of annihilation. In practice, we can use the *Kleshas* as a reference point for our feelings about any given experience. Are we feeling drawn toward or away from something (*raga* and *dwesha*)? Are we resisting the experience we are in because it challenges how we see ourselves (*Asmitā*)? Are we refusing to see the bigger picture (*Avidyā*)? Are we terrified of the unknown (*Abhinivesha*)? If we understand the cause of our affliction, then we can determine whether it is aligned with want, desire, or longing. Then we can choose how to meet it accordingly.

In a feeling-averse culture like our own, choosing to feel and respond is a bold commitment as well as a huge risk. To acknowledge the stir of emotion rather than suppress it may feel like losing control, but we can work with these stirrings by recognizing them as the gateway to surrender. When we enter into the tender and vulnerable space of experience, every experience, we learn to face whatever arises. This is the space of longing: open, vulnerable, perilous, and true. It is oriented inward and centered on the recognition of our own essential presence as part of something much bigger, much more profound, and understanding that to serve, honor, and respect that bigger thing does *not* require our personal diminishment. This is an act of extreme bravery in a culture that teaches us that playing small is the same as humility, that service is equated with self-sacrifice, and that perfection is the only thing worth striving for.

Navigating the unfamiliar waters of emotion is an ability that can be learned, an instrument that can be sharpened. With time and practice, we can come to see our emotion as another form of intelligence that we can wield with skill in our lives, and we can engage with each occurrence as such. We become less afraid to feel what arises and develop a deepening curiosity about the ways our feelings and emotions are communicating and guiding us. We take our sentiments and sensitivities out of "time out" and learn to provide the necessary space for them to be seen, heard, respected, and heeded.

Through this recalibration of our relationship with our emotions, we become less bound by our histories, traumas, and patterns and more interested in the impetus that is driving us. Our wants become opportunities to explore what compels us. As we become closer to owning ourselves fully, our desires become fuel for our actions and the gifts we offer, and our longings become our solace, our touchpoints that keep us plugged into a bigger picture of space, time, and history. We feel less shaken and impacted by the actions and choices of others, less guarded in our engagement. We become resilient.

Resilience and Healing

The tools and concepts of healing and trauma are beyond my scope of expertise. However, when we explore and experience resilience, healing unfolds. Want is often a call for healing with a perfectly valid and purposeful voice. But, because it is fueled by lack, it may take us away from our potential to expand and toward the deepening of our wounded parts. Want reinforces our disconnection from having and our connection to not having. And, unfortunately, obtaining the object of our want rarely satisfies the hunger that we seek to eliminate. The Buddhist teachings call this the realm of "hungry ghosts." The concept is that we can easily be tormented by our lack of things and driven to "insatiable desire, hunger or thirst as a result of bad deeds" (TDB, "Hungry Ghosts," n.p.). From a Yogic perspective, these "bad deeds" are experiences that originate from our ignorance (*Avidyā*), which lead us to strengthen our identification (*asmita*), our attachments (*Rāga*), and our aversions (*dwesha*). Without awareness, we are destined to repeat these same cycles of wanting, gaining, and dissatisfaction in perpetuity, finding that no amount of wealth, love, stuff, or support can really ever provide the outcomes we seek.

Author and psychologist Esther Perel asserts that "desire is to own the wanting" and that this can only be done by a "sovereign self that is free to choose." And that is "why desire is so intimately connected with a sense of self-worth" (Tippett, "Esther Perel," n p.). To recognize our desires as opposed to our wants is to see the guideposts to our own value and authority, and it is essential to our freedom. When we deny our desires, we are working not only to separate ourselves from that which is bigger than us but also from our own inner yearning. Desire turns us toward the voice that allows us to calibrate our compass arrows inward and attune ourselves to self-trust. When we sever our connection to our desires, Yoga says, we are wandering in a fog. We are lost and misguided. The truest way to return to the clarity of your path is to turn toward the deepest pull from inside and act from that place.

Practice and Application

Feel and Observe: Call to mind something that you really want, a goal that you are still working toward. Observe the feelings that arise in your body and breath as you contemplate this. Now, call to mind a feeling of desire, different from want; it feels more like a calling, something you feel that you *are* rather than something you want to obtain, achieve, or complete. Observe the feelings that arise in body and breath. Finally, seek out a feeling of longing, a pull, an immersion. Observe how the experience of this feeling is translated to your body and breath.

Inquiry: What is your deepest driving desire? How does it express itself in and through your commitments, your actions, and words?

Movement: Begin in child's pose. With eyes closed, touch the tenderness of your desire or longing. Breathe into that place and feeling inside. Allow whatever surfaces to arise (emotion, vocalization, movement), and follow its lead. Slowly begin to move in any way that this tender desire or longing within is inspiring you to move. Feel that your movements are making more space for your desire to inhabit the container of your body. Put music on if it helps. Cover your eyes if you need to. Use this time to engage with your inner desires and longings without the distraction of the external world.

Āsana and Energetics Suggestions:
Explore these āsanas *as a force of stabilization and renewal* (prāṇa).

CRP
Setu Bandha Sarvāṅgāsana
Adho Mukha Śhvānāsana
Utkatāsana
Parivṛtta Pārśhvakoṇāsana
Ardha Matsyendrāsana
Śhavāsana

10

The Wound

An elder I greatly admire refers to the dominant culture of North America as the "walking wounded." Scroll through any social media platform, and this observation would be a difficult point to argue against.

In the last few years, it has become "sexy" to display our wounds, to create sets of requirements around them, and to roll out a list of expectations for others to meet in order for our tender and delicate parts to be protected and honored. Though the sentiment is worthy and perhaps even warranted, the system that has been built around these ideas is profoundly contributing to our lack of resilience and leading us further and further away from our innate state and the experience of Yoga.

As we become more focused on excavating and understanding our wounds, there is a danger of overidentifying with what we unearth as the whole of who we are, which can lead to inaccurate self-definition. This tendency is the primary thing that Yoga works to prevent and that resilience allows us to expand beyond. When we define ourselves by our wounds, we begin to see ourselves as fragile and incapable of risk. We can become dependent on others to make our world safe and require those around us to create the perfect conditions for us to thrive.

To be clear, I do vehemently agree that suffering and oppression need acknowledgment and that accountability is imperative, but as with most things, the slope is slippery and can easily cycle back into the all-too-familiar systems of power and impunity. The result is that we may be becoming a culture that commodifies and identifies with trauma, trauma that is exacerbated and exploited by many of the approaches that claim to heal it. The self-help industry is becoming a monster in its own right, demanding and tormenting, recreating the cycle of victimhood and oppression from the very desire to heal and be healed. This supposition might be "triggering" to those who are deeply committed to healing the wounds of the past, both individual and collective. And I want to state that I very much believe in the necessity of healing, but the wound is an aspect of self that is both essential and powerful from a Yogic point of view. And it's time we broach the subject with courage as well as care, not just for the wounded individual or community but also for the story that extends before and beyond this lifetime. So here I go, diving into the frenzy of the walking wounded and daring to speak my mind.

Everyone is wounded. Every. One. Yes, our wounds vary in degrees and severity across time and culture, but the impacts of our individual wounds are severe and traumatic to each of us in a way that is a fallacy to compare or disregard. Because our individual wounds are essential pieces to our unique story that cannot be cast aside, regardless of their origin, they are impacting every aspect of our lived experience and rippling outward in ways that we may not even realize. Similar to the provocations regarding dichotomy in Chapter 6, this tendency to sort our individual wounds in order to create a hierarchy of trauma might be at the core of our collective problems.

Yoga does not teach that we are without wounds, nor does it guide us to be wound-free at the culmination of our practice. It does not provide a road map for avoiding wounds or a shield from the devastations that this life inevitably brings. And that is a blessing that many struggle, and even refuse, to permit. Yoga does not advocate solely for positivity or optimism and quite directly argues against attempting to bypass pain and instead asks us to join with it. Yoga calls on us to understand our afflictions as a necessary part of the divine design and to have the willpower to sustain that design and, at the highest levels of practice, to be fully present in our woes in a way that releases our identification of pain with suffering. Yoga characterizes all the ways we are (and continue to be) wounded as a strength rather than a weakness. From a Yogic point of view, we practice in order to access the strength that is ever available within and from our pain.

We Are Wired for This: Understanding Vāsanā and Samskāra

Healing our wounds has become of paramount importance and for good reason. Yoga says that our bodies are a storehouse of our experiences, all of which leave impressions on our breath, the energetic transformer of our bodies. We are, according to Yoga, literally a composite of wounds and vitality and tendencies to be wounded as well as vitalized. This isn't an accident; it's access. According to Yoga, we are born with certain in-built patterns that engage us in specific types of outcomes.

92

10. The Wound

"*Samskāra*" in Sanskrit means the subtle mental impressions left by all thoughts, intentions, and actions that an individual has ever experienced. Often likened to grooves in the mind, they can be viewed as psychological or emotional imprints that contribute to the formation of behavioral patterns. *Samskāras* are below the level of normal consciousness and are said to be the root of all impulses, character traits, and innate dispositions.

Samskāra is derived from the Sanskrit word "*sam*," which means "well planned," and "*kar*," which means "the action that is taken." The idea of Samskāra is that we have an innate structure of response and action that is "well planned" and strategic and will help us to learn, grow, and evolve. These plans are free of the dichotomy of good or bad and right or wrong and lead us to make choices that serve the lessons we are created to learn. We can become skillful in the understanding of *Samskāra* when we begin to apply the knowledge and experience of our past actions to our present moments. This choice is called "*Viveka*" in Sanskrit, which means "discernment."

Because we are wired for certain individual actions based on our past impressions (as well as the contracts we are born with, known as "*Karma*"), we have tendencies toward certain behaviors in our lives. These tendencies are known as "*Vāsanā*." "*Vāsanā*" refers to a past impression in the mind that influences behavior. *Vāsanās*, like *samskāras*, are not innately good or bad and instead play an essential role in how we individuate from the whole of things through our experiences, responses, and reactions.

Sumskāra and Vāsanā

"*Samskara*" also means "activator" in Sanskrit. It is the subtle imprint that leaves its mark on the subconscious and unconscious mind. A *Samskāra* is an impression left by an original experience (be it positive or negative) that spun off into behavioral responses, habits, patterns, and even protections. We can have a *Samskāra* of a positive experience, such as "I said thank you, and my mom acknowledged it with words of praise," or negative, like "I touched the hot stove, and it was very painful." *Samskāras* can also be indirect and not so easily identifiable beyond the subconscious and unconscious patterns of the mind. When activated, *samskāras* result in *vāsanās*, the aforementioned behavioral responses, habits, patterns, and protections that result from the initial impression. Examples of *vāsanās* at play look like "I always use impeccable manners in order to receive praise and validation" or "I avoid taking risks because when I do, I always get hurt/burned."

Saṃskāras and *vāsanās* work together to create patterns of behavior and if left unchecked can become a "runaway train" of reactions and responses over which we seem to have no control. When we allow our behavior to bypass review, we miss the opportunity to learn what lessons that *Saṃskāra* and *Vāsanā* provide. We feel unable to use the tool of *Viveka* to assess and distinguish our reactions, and we forgo our ability to choose our responses.

Perhaps the most confounding power of *Saṃskāra* and *Vāsanā* is the way they seem to act against our better judgment and despite the quiet whisper of our inner voice telling us that we are out of alignment with ourselves. Because *Saṃskāra* and *Vāsanā* are learned and expressed behaviors, they are often reinforced by our external environment and validated over and over again by voices that are not our own. Many, though not all, *saṃskāras* and *vāsanās* apply strategies to disregard our deepest driving desires in order to serve the learned and expected behavior of others, including society as a whole. This creates a quiet but undeniable dissonance between our own inner voice and our outer expectations, which began in our youth and became so habituated throughout life that we lost our connection to the quiet whispers of our heart.

How to Work with the Wound

As we work to identify the impressions and experiences that have left their mark upon our individual expression, we desire to "heal" what we discover, a process that is often characterized by more discovery of more wounds, requiring more healing in a cycle that never ceases. Sometimes we become entrenched in the process of "healing" all the broken parts of ourselves only to find that each trauma is a doorway to the next. In seeking to remedy the pain of our past and protect our future selves from having to repeat the process, we withdraw from the living that our aliveness calls us toward. Somewhere along the way, healing has become associated with safety and the act of self-perfecting and, in many ways, prevents the wounded from living life until the healing is complete. Though the process of healing is as unique and individual as the wounded person themselves, it is not independent of living. Learning how to integrate healing into the lived experience of the here and now, to accept what is both within and without and willingly move

94

into it is what being resilient is all about. Rather than tapping out, resilience is an invitation to step in with all the tender and scarred parts and choose to keep turning into the hairpin turns that life offers despite the risk.

So much of the work of healing calls us back into our bodies, a place that many in the dominant culture of North America have abandoned. Healing work can look like *āsana*, *prāṇāyāma*, meditation, or Yoga, as well as professional forms of therapy. It can also look like walking in the woods or speaking your mind. Often unbeknownst to us is our bodies' immense capacity to heal and thrive despite even the deepest of wounds. When we choose the body as an access point to healing, we reconnect with the wellspring of our aliveness, the fountain of our vital energy and life force. When we access the body and the breath, healing is simple (though not easy), but it is complicated by our mental attachment and identification to our wounds that keep us re-traumatizing ourselves over and over. In order to access the healing capacity of our dynamic system, we must allow for our own resilience to emerge. We must create the opportunity to engage with the unknown, to make mistakes, and to be hurt again and again, rather than continually pulling away from the risk that may also be (and often is) the pathway to reward. It's our identification with trauma, our necessity to be seen and understood and cared for within the context of our trauma, that keeps us from truly healing in a way that makes us resilient, makes life buoyant, and makes Yoga accessible.

Yoga works by directly asking us to connect with the part of us that is deeper than the mind in order to recognize and be in a relationship with our tendencies of identification. The deeper practices entreat us to really understand ourselves from within and to discern what parts of our behavior we desire to keep and what parts we are ready to release. The challenge then becomes the application of our agency and power of choice regarding whether to continue to identify as we have in the past or make a change.

Resilience offers a similar challenge. It invites us to recognize that a world without wounds is a world without empathy, compassion, humility, lessons, and growth. Though it seems that we all want it, a wound-free world lacks depth, flavor, and maturity. Our wounds make us rich: they are the fodder of our lives. Though they may be tragic and traumatic, they are also the threshold that we must cross for our own evolution. Our wounds are our initiation—unique and often cruel but necessary for our individual expression of self. Our wounds are essential to our self-definition, and when viewed through the lens of resilience, they can simply be a part of our dynamic and complex story rather than the whole of it. A wound-centric approach that demands healing to occur before life can truly be lived often exchanges the beauty that fills our days with a perpetual engagement with our pain and suffering to the point that it clouds our sight. This cycle can become habitual and feel comfortable in its familiarity, allowing our minds to recreate the trauma in ourselves over and over again, long after the body has healed. When we choose to accept our wounds as a part of who we are—"warts and all," as they say—and work to integrate them as a part of our whole self, then we have begun the Yogic alchemy of transforming our wounds into the weapons we wield in the world, ultimately providing access to our vitality, our power, and our purpose.

Practice and Application

Feel and Observe: Take a moment to recall a painful incident or experience. Observe where and how this memory feels inside your body. Observe how even the memory expresses itself through your breath. Though it is hard, stay with the feelings that arose. Do your best not to let your mind run away with the story and instead stay with the thoughts or memory only enough to generate the feelings in your body. What happens when you stay with the feelings? Observe the process. Does it change after a bit of time passes? Does it intensify or diminish? Feel only as long as you are able to, then take a short walk or jump up and down to release any residual discomfort from the process.

Inquiry: What are my wounds? How do they express themselves in my life?

Movement: Make sure your space is clear of obstacles. Recall the feelings you initiated in the Feel and Observe section (if you haven't done that yet, please do it now). As the feelings surface, begin to "lean in" to them. Physically move your body in the direction of the internal sensations. If you feel the desire to shout or scream or cry, do it. Feel the intensity of the feelings you have called up and allow that intensity to move through your physical form. Maybe you shake, maybe you stomp, maybe you spin around in circles, maybe you punch the air. Trust your body's impulses. Keep following the body's suggestions to make space for all the power that these feelings and memories hold. Lean in little by little at first, right up to the razor's edge of intensity, then back off. With continued practice, the razor's edge will soften, and you will gain access to the immensity of power that lies within you.

10. The Wound

Āsana and Energetics Suggestions:
Explore these āsanas *as a path to unfold understanding, empathy, and* acceptance (apāna).

CRP
Bālāsana
Adho Mukha Śhvānāsana
Uttānāsana
Prasārita Pādottānāsana
Legs Up the Wall
Śhavāsana

11

The Weapon

In the practice of Yoga, we work to identify our "weaknesses" through inquiry and to understand, accept, and integrate them. In doing so, we convert the wounded, traumatized parts of ourselves (quite consciously) into our points of strength. This process necessarily requires us to bring all our broken and wounded parts with us on the journey of a life well lived, regardless of where we are in the process of healing. It is a process of alchemizing our pain and trauma in a way that "yokes" us to our past and supports us as we move into the future. It challenges us to engage with our lives fully without the demand for perfection (either of the past or future) and encourages us to bring the lessons of our wounds with us as we meet each new, though often familiar, experience. In this way, our wound becomes the weapon that we can wield skillfully as we meet our lives face forward.

This approach does not require perfection nor a predictable outcome. It does not demand positivity or happiness. It does not require the external world to align to our feelings of safety or validate our path. It does make us fully responsible for ourselves. It calls on us to recognize the role we play in our victimhood and to be accountable for the feelings and responses that arise from our wounds. It demands of us the courage to act with conscious engagement, compelling us to acknowledge and feel, and to be skillful in response to what we discover. Alchemizing the wound into the weapon provides space for the truth of our pain and difficulty without feeding feelings of resistance to it. It can be most closely related to the ideas of surrender that we explored in Chapters 7 and 8—it is an action not of release but of reclamation.

Weapon

The word itself may be "activating" for some of us. A weapon connotes danger, power, strength, and fear. In the Yogic pantheon, all the deities are depicted with weapons in their many hands. More accurately referred to as attributes, these weapons are representations that vary based on the symbology of each deity and are used to describe the deities' qualities rather than define them. The weapons that each deity possesses are examples of the power that they can wield. Though these weapons may be used for purposes of destruction or even pain, the same weapons have the power to transform, to liberate, and to be of benefit. The weapons are the symbol of each deity's unique power and prowess and the reason that we would turn toward that specific deity when guidance or support is needed.

Take the goddess Durga, for example. She is often represented in anthropomorphic form with ten arms, each holding a different weapon that represent her attributes of power, fearlessness, dignity, and invincibility. In her hands, she carries the weapons of all the gods as well as a lotus and a conch shell. Her sword (*khanda*) signifies the intellectual sharpness of discrimination (*Viveka*), and her thunderbolt represents steadfastness, will, and determination (*icchā shakti*). Each weapon, including the benign ones, has a particular significance related to the power of the one who holds them. In the same way, our own weapons give us a spectrum of allocations from strength and perseverance to courage and compassion.

When we come to understand that every wound and scar is an access point to our own personal power and understanding, then Yoga begins. When we dare to yoke ourselves to our pain rather than remedy it, healing is what results. Rather than wish our pain and wounds away, we can harness the experiences of our own suffering and digest them as pieces of our unique story. We begin to see that all we have endured has shaped us, turned us, polished us like gemstones, despite the damage and suffering it may have caused. With time and commitment, we can bring forth the spectrum of each experience that expands beyond the experience itself and offers us the opportunity to give our content context. This process takes patience and time, but with practice, it becomes more efficient and more effective.

Touching the wound to access the power of the weapon doesn't mean making the pain and trauma positive. It doesn't mean that what didn't kill us made us stronger. It simply means that what didn't kill us made us. Maybe it made us more cautious, calmer, or more creative. Maybe it gave us access to empathy or rage. Maybe it expanded our capacity for joy. Whatever the wound provided, it is a part of our story, and the only way to find power from it is to claim it. When we are faced with our own pain, we often desire to eliminate or annihilate it because to hold it is so uncomfortable, but the practice of transforming suffering into strength requires a capacity to sustain that discomfort.

It's not so dissimilar in our physical bodies. When we desire our muscles to become stronger or more flexible, we must tear them little by little, and we must endure the intensity of the process and the time it takes to mend the tears with new tissue, which equates to strength and length. We cannot grow our physical capacity and strength without being wounded first. Resilience isn't the product of the absence of difficulty; it is the direct result of it. When we begin to see our difficulties as resources rather than defects, then we are in Yoga and in the process of resilience.

One of the pitfalls of this alchemizing process is that it is happening perpetually whether or not we realize it. Our reactivity, our "trigger responses," our defensiveness, our posturing are all sourced in our wounds and pain, and these reactions are all happening all the time, even if we are blind to it. "Until you make the unconscious conscious, it will direct your life and you will call it fate" (Jung, "Until You," n.p.).

Bringing our awareness to the parts of ourselves that are hard to see is the most difficult aspect of transforming the wound into the weapon. Our unrecognized pain and suffering are the very source of our ammunition in the world. We are weaponizing our pain and our desire to protect ourselves from its recurrence all the time. But when we choose to bring our awareness, our agency, and our choice into the process, the use of our weapon becomes graceful and even helpful. This is the proposition of a Yoga practice: to yoke ourselves to our pain and difficulty so that we can access the energy and power contained within our suffering. Once we can do that, transforming our wounds into our weapons is a process of skill and refinement. By choosing to be in a relationship with the wounded and unsavory parts of ourselves, we can bring awareness to how we express them in our experiences both with ourselves and with others in the world and choose how we desire to use them.

When we resist the work of self-inquiry and reflection, we resist the requirement of being accountable for our responses and our actions, whether or not they are sourced from our woundedness or our healing. Awareness and consciousness provide a lens through which we can view our responses and reactions with agency and discernment. We can work to make our choices, reactions, and responses conscious rather than involuntary. And they do not have to be perfect. From skillfulness, we wield our weapons with intent, understanding that each swing and blow generates consequences.

11. The Weapon

Surrender Is a Luxury Until It Becomes a Necessity

When discussions of wound work come up, they are usually cloaked in hooks of identity and denial. Owning our role in the continuation of our pain is an additional level of devastation that we must endure, and for those who have been or are continuing to endure traumatic and difficult experiences or whose identity is intimately connected to the wound, it can feel like a threat to our very being. To become accountable for our attachment to our wounds, to acknowledge our own comfort with our habitual responses, to question ourselves and to recognize our contribution to our own struggle can feel like a betrayal to our very being. This can cause us to act in accord with the familiarity of our pain, protecting ourselves by staying safely behind the curtain of our past experiences. This can cause us to assume that all our experiences are guaranteed to repeat themselves and be willfully ignorant to the ways that we contribute to our own suffering. Eventually, either from exhaustion, additional trauma, illness, or loss, we may surrender to our experience and begin to see the part we play in the story. This surrender, which results in a refusal to weave a narrative of excuse and enabling, provides an access point to the awareness necessary to transform our pain into our power.

The work of Yoga and resilience is to engage and support surrender before we reach the proverbial rock bottom. When we can surrender to what is, as it is, when it is, and recognize our contribution to it, we can adjust and adapt in the very moment of our emerging awareness based on our discernment. We can hold the wounded parts of ourselves with tenderness as the pain and fear surface and make choices on how we will direct what we are seeing and feeling rather than be swept away by it. In the work of somatic healing, this requires deep assessment and understanding of bodily responses, which include long buried tensions, anxieties, and patterns. This work, when approached and explored separately from the moments of extreme trauma responses hijacking our agency, can be a luxury.

Surrendering into the truth of what is happening now is possible in every moment and does not require extreme difficulty or an overwhelming situation to force our hand. When surrender is a luxury, it provides a stable foundation from which we can approach the more unexpected and challenging troubles. Remember that the practice of surrender is often referred to in modern Yoga lexicon as "letting go" and is not a simple nor straightforward process. As we have explored for several chapters, we can never truly be "free" of difficulty and pain, but we can be "free" within it. And this freedom is our resilience; it is the experience of Yoga.

So many of the ancient texts of Yoga express that surrender is the supreme goal. It is an experience or release that is more closely related to letting in than ridding ourselves of anything. It is an allowance of what is, in its entirety, and the willingness to see it in a larger context. Surrender removes the veils and hooks of our self-denial and defense and places us squarely in the center of our experience. It provides the space for things to "not be okay" and holds in tandem "what it could be." Surrender is *not* the will to desire a situation to change, regardless of our external circumstances or the pain it causes. In practice, it lets go of nothing but our want for things to be different than they are.

Thus, surrender is a luxury until it is a necessity. Eventually, we will all have an experience of loss, grief, or trauma during which denial is not available to us or there is no one to defend against. From heartbreak, to death, to violence, to the incessant tedium of a life ignored, every human being will have the opportunity to surrender as a necessity. Even if the opportunity is missed or overlooked through practices of numbing or denial, the experiences are far from forgotten and will continue to surface in repeating patterns of greater and greater degrees of difficulty and distress. I often tell my students that the invitation to surrender comes in a quiet whisper that inevitably grows to a shout and culminates in a slap across the face (or, as a student recently pointed out, you will be dragged kicking and screaming), but however it comes, come it will. The practice of Yoga and resilience is to learn to hear the invitation at the level of the whisper (a luxury) and to respond skillfully to it in the hopes that we may avert being dragged.

When we ignore the whisper and wait for the shout, slap, or drag to respond to the invitation, we may find ourselves in situations of devastation and disorientation to such a degree that ignorance is not an option and for which we have no tools or weapons to easily employ. An absence of understanding and a surplus of armor create conditions for surrender in which our choice is minimal and our autonomy is distant.

These places are often called "crises" and can be internal or external (or both at once). And they are inevitable. Neither Yoga nor resilience nor unending positivity and optimism can protect our humanness from our own frailty, but both Yoga and resilience can provide a life raft on which to rest and catch our breath between the rising and crashing waves of life. Crises are real, sometimes extreme, and as unique as the individual themselves. And they are a part of the design of our human life. They are not a

malfunction; they are an invitation. Contained within them are the building blocks of maturity and growth, of our personal power and our realization of our place in a bigger picture. Crises are the grounds for resilience
that call forth the opportunity for our wounds to become our weapons on
the battlefield of surrender.

In these moments, we begin to reclaim our liability as our biggest
asset, and rather than hide or protect our vulnerabilities, we move to
engage with them in honest and clear conversation. This is the process of
transforming the wound into the weapon With the bedrock of attenuation and assimilation, we can boldly choose to integrate our pain and suffering into the whole of who we are and, in doing so, source the power that
supports us in sustaining, enduring, and recovering from challenge and
difficulty.

How Do We Transform Our Wound into Our Weapon?

There is no one way to access the power and support available to each
of us via the portal of our unique individual pain, but there are some general guidelines to work with in the process. Most of these are anecdotal
and therefore specific to the situations that they address, but I will try to
offer generalized conclusions that will help you to see how these principles
can be applied to a spectrum of wounds.

All of us have residual pain, shame, and trauma from our upbring-
ing. Even if we had the most loving and supportive environment during
our formative years, we are bound to carry little breaks and tears inside
acquired from the necessary separation that comes with growing up.
Some of the most common wounds are around worth and value and
enoughness. Many wounded adults hold within them the deep cuts of
unworthiness, low value, and not enoughness that were a felt response
to some external feedback that may or may not have intended the result.
Regardless of the motive, our small children's minds interpreted our
adult and environmental feedback as problems that needed to be solved
or corrected in order for us to retain the love and care we require for
survival.

In the Tantric tradition, the primary wounds that underlie our blindness to our true limitless Self are called "*malas*" (pronounced muh-luh,
rather than mālā). "*Mala*" means "impurity," and it's the universal dust
on the lens. *Mala* manifests as fundamental experiences of disconnection
from the bigger picture (i.e., the scope of time, history, future potential,

true self) and leaves us with a sense of being incomplete no matter the genuineness of our pursuits.

The three *malas* are: *Ānava mala*—the fundamental sense of lack; *māyīya mala*—the fundamental sense of being separate; and *Karma mala*—the fundamental sense that we alone are the doer. This teaching addresses the inevitable wounds that all humans must endure. The *malas* point us to the recognition that our struggles are human ones, though they often feel as if they are only happening to us. It also calls on us to remember that the practices of Yoga and resilience do not teach us to avoid or deny these wounds but rather to recognize them and bring consciousness to the choices we make when they arise.

These wounds are most evident in the modes of protection in our day-to-day lives as adults. Contrary to our true desires, our wounds live in constant fear of being reinforced and run outdated (and often inappropriate) strategies to keep us safe (called "*Vikalpa*" or "contrary intention" in Sanskrit). In the case of feelings of unworthiness, our wounds might have us running around at the expense of our own health and safety to provide for the needs of others (at work, at home, and in our relationships). We come to believe that if we don't prove our worth all the time, then those that we value will judge us as unworthy of love and leave us behind. Our wounds react to the smallest of oversights, processing them through our habituated patterns of perception as evidence of our unworthiness; therefore, we scurry around faster and with more concern about rejection, attempting to show our value and all the while deepening the wound within.

We can never receive enough validation to "heal" our wounded parts (after all, they are a part of the design), so we repeat and increase the patterns over and over again. Until we are able to recognize these patterns, we will continue to recreate the opportunities for them to be seen. For example, once we are able to see our own engagement in our wounds of unworthiness, we are able to hold our wounded parts in a space of compassionate understanding. Reconciliation and reclamation of our exiled parts take place when we do the work of honoring and allowing the wounds to exist and calling forth compassion and integration instead of removal. When we see our patterns of protection from the eyes of the child trying to do their best to hold on to the love that was essential for their survival, and we can cry or scream or love in the way that our wounded child was unable to do, then we are capturing the power contained in those wounds. This gives us the choice as to how we want to use that power. Acknowledgment of our exiled parts begins the process of returning them back into the space of the whole and reuniting with our forgotten and lost pieces of self.

This powerful act of recognition is the catalyst for resolving the false understandings that have kept us separate from the full capacity of who we are. As we call back the wounded parts, we begin to forgive our shortcomings and be compassionate toward ourselves during the moments in which our pain was running the show. That reclamation is the source of a newfound awareness that empowers us to protect ourselves when necessary, but it also creates the possibility of expanding our threshold of risk and growing our capacity to handle such risk. It is this alchemy of turning our wound into our weapon that gives us access to greater possibility and greater capacity.

The realization that the pain we feel contains the very power we seek is the turning point on our path of Yoga and resilience. When we stop refusing our pain and use the feelings, emotions, thoughts, and sensations as an entryway to awareness of our power, we are transforming our wound into our weapon. It is the wound of our unworthiness that can provide the inspiration to put down the burden of proving our worth and to be present with and as the one who is already worthy, loved, and understood. This weapon of worth, arising from the wound of our unworthiness, might direct us to a painting class instead of meal planning or into meditation rather than overscheduling. And in doing so, not only will we set ourselves free to be who and as we are, but also our frenzied behavior that affects those around us will calm down. When we stop trying to provide for everyone else's needs, we give space for those around us to discover their own agency and choice and step into their own autonomy as well.

Practice and Application

Feel and Observe: Be still and quiet. Observe the strategies you use to protect yourself from your own wounds. Feel your personal experience of lack in your body and what physical, mental, and emotional responses engage to protect you. Feel your personal experience of separation, and notice how your entire system responds to the threat of being separate. Feel your wound of being all on your own to solve your problems and soothe your pain. Sense how this loneliness expresses itself. Observe how all these pain points have contributed to the creation of strategies of protection.

Inquiry: What weapons are hidden in your wounds? How are you already alchemizing your pain to be your power? Are you doing it in the way that you want? Are there awarenesses and skills that you can bring to bear to refine this transformation?

Movement: With music (or silently), begin to move with abandon. Take up a lot of space; make a lot of noise. Flail, fling, growl, howl. Be wild. Feel the wildness in you expressing itself through movement. Slowly begin to soothe this wild part of yourself. Give it space and tenderness. Allow it to run itself out until it is anchored. Feel the power that once felt out of control begin expressing itself in and through you with more grace and ease. Continue to move until you feel called to a natural conclusion. Land in the still point of full integration. Take a moment to be there.

Āsana and Energetics Suggestions:

Explore these āsanas *as a means to empower and strengthen your discoveries (*samāna).

Tadāsana
Utkatāsana
Uttānāsana
Nāvāsana
Setu Bandha Sarvāṅgāsana
Śhavāsana

12

The Art of Critical Thought

The transformation of the wound into the weapon teaches us that we are more resilient when we are sovereign. From the place of "owning ourselves fully," to paraphrase van der Kolk (*The Body Keeps the Score*), we access a wellspring of inner trust and confidence, we are more connected, more available, more present, and more buoyant. When we experience this freedom and trust, we are in the experience of Yoga every day and in as many moments as possible. We are independent yet connected; we are strong yet soft. We are confident yet willing to yield, bend, and stretch to learn more, to evolve, and to open up to greater possibility.

Opening up to more is the essence of a resilient life, one of which we choose to meet our experiences as they present themselves and trust that we have the tools to adapt, adjust, and expand as necessary. It is a rebellious process of allowing what *is* to be true and daring to step into whatever we find wherever we find it without the requirements of our safety, approval, or certainty. When we open up to each moment, whether good or bad, we allow a bigger truth to emerge. We stretch the boundaries of our limited perspectives and create space to receive more than we thought possible. In our opening, we grow our capacity, little by little at first and then by leaps and bounds, not only to endure the difficulties that life unrelentingly hands us but also to immerse in the simple and profound beauty of being alive. We are able to walk in the world with shattered hearts, heavy disappointments, persistent conflicts, and even great loss without losing sight of the joy that is also present in the most seemingly insignificant expressions. So much is expressed in every bud and bloom, even as they die away, becoming the ground, the air, and the space that we occupy.

In contrast, when we move from a place of protection, we often diminish our potential and become stuck in our ingrained patterns of behavior and belief. We can become unwilling to question our current modes of understanding and often reduce our opportunities to grow beyond our present state. When we are unwilling to learn, to look, to wonder, and to be curious, we opt to reinforce our existing beliefs rather than expand or change them. We find ourselves seeking out the experiences in life that reflect and support our resistance, inertia, or attachment without contemplating whether or not the experiences are harmful or helpful. We may limit our capacity to consider new or different ideas as well as the ideas and opinions of others. This reduction of capacity and willingness is often directly correlated to a disinclination for critical thought, especially when related to self-reflection, and leads us to the repetition of dysfunction over and over again.

Unwillingness to apply critique to our own thoughts and reflections can have myriad sources. Perhaps it's because we don't trust ourselves due to past experiences or feedback and judgment from others. Perhaps we feel most comfortable with what is familiar and therefore accept it as correct. Perhaps questioning ourselves and others feels too threatening to our identities and to the tenuous status quo. Whatever the reason, unless we are driven to reflect on the situations and circumstances in which we find ourselves, the task is largely ignored. Even when invited to reflect upon our habitual thoughts, actions, and patterns of behavior, resistance is often at the forefront with the intention of preventing us from embarking on any reflection that would put us in the seat of being wrong or mistaken. This resistance to critical thinking is a prime symptom of the absence of resilience and the inability to be fully accountable for our engagement and to reflect on our own actions as well as on the actions and choices of others.

Critical thought about ourselves and our world is at the core of our sovereignty. The art of inquiring about our identity, probing our personal perspective, and alchemizing our wounds lead us to discover a foundation rooted in something deeper than the external past, culture, rules, or expectations. When we access confidence, inner trust, and willingness to open up rather than close and restrict, we are in prime territory for the courageous undertaking of critical thought: daring to question what we know. The process of critical thinking liberates us from the need to prove or defend our belief systems and instead invites us to become infinitely curious about how the world works and our engagement with it. We become enthralled by the mechanisms of action and interaction both within and outside of us. We no longer make assumptions about the truth of things. Instead, we inquire, we wonder, we probe. We dare to question ourselves and the world. Our queries may lead us to discoveries of the ways we were misinterpreting situations based on false understanding, which is the essence of empathy. They may also show us that what we thought was "wrong" is simply different, and they may challenge us to change our minds. The latter possibility, though liberating, is often the most threatening of all.

In our modern culture, changing our minds is often seen as weakness or instability, and so we struggle to provoke the possibility within ourselves. Shifting our beliefs or understandings has moved from the realm of intelligence to the arena of condemnation, and given the current political climate, this stance is not poised to change anytime soon. The threat of being outcast poses a substantial challenge to the application of critical thought. In cultivating a willingness to see things differently than we originally did, we risk being expelled from the groups and memberships that have offered us a sense of belonging. Changing perspective is the precursor to changing our minds, which jeopardizes our inclusion in the groups in which our identity is upheld. In recent years, changing our minds has become synonymous with "flip-flopping" and is criticized harshly. Culturally, we are expected to "know" what's right and wrong with very little leeway given to the actual process of learning and experimentation and with almost no allowance for the learning that comes from mistakes and amendment. So, in the world of resilience, the capacity to think critically—to question what we "know" and to be curious about what we are told, to dare to think about the nature of things—is a fragile art, and it's a revolutionary act.

The goal of critical thinking is not to determine a right or wrong conclusion but to explore the innumerable possibilities that exist between the dichotomies. To wonder about the way things are and ponder about the way things could be are the capacities it offers. The point of critical thought, whether explored alone or in the company of others, is not to discover answers but rather to become open to deeper and deeper levels of questioning and curiosity, to peel back the layers of the known, and to be open to what could be discovered. Critical thought, though rarely taught, has been a valued system of discourse since antiquity, and its results were never predicated on agreement. As Stephen Greenblatt reflects in his book, *The Swerve*, ancient conversation and debate did not have the purpose of determination, but rather

> the exchange itself, not its final conclusions, carries much of the meaning. The discussion itself is what most matters, the fact that we can reason together easily, with a blend of wit and seriousness, never descending into gossip or slander and always allowing room for alternative views [p. 70].

In Yoga, this practice of inquiry is called "*vichara*," and the discoveries we make provide the tools for discernment and choice "*Viveka*." The ability to be discerning in our choices is essential to the process of evolution and growth. The determination and willpower (*icchā shakti*) to question what we believe and what we are told make up the bedrock of sovereignty. They make us fully accountable for our actions and require us to reflect on how the results of our decisions impact not only our individual experience but also the widening circles of the collective. Critical thought, when applied without the condition of perfection or correction, allows us to explore diverse perspectives, contemplate potential outcomes, question consequences, and to stretch beyond our small zone of sight and into more collaborative understanding.

The stickiness of critical thought isn't actually in the criticism itself but in the way it has been applied for so long. If we can shift our common interpretation of critique to something more closely related to its original intent and learn to use critical thinking differently, critique can become the power to expand our knowledge and ultimately to change the world. In classical Greek and Roman discourse, the point was never to agree but instead to exchange views, which often resulted in inconclusive outcomes yet created the opportunity for each participant in the conversation to expand their individual understanding and polish their position. Inquiry can lead to deeper levels of understanding and self-recognition. It can result in accountability and repair, and it can guide us to be more aligned with our core values and our beliefs and bring integrity to our actions in the world. More than anything else, the cultivation of critical thought can teach us how to anchor trust inwardly by providing access to a knowledge that is inherent and independent of outside influence.

Critical Thought and Trust

Trusting that our inner knowing is worth heeding gives us the capacity to choose what is right for us without the demand that it is right for everyone and ultimately to accept the unique perspectives of the world that color our existence. As a child, my parents called this inner knowing "conscience"; as an adult, I've come to know it as autonomy. It expresses itself as curiosity, challenge, inquiry, and questioning. It compels us to know ourselves more deeply rather than only to seek our reflection in the eyes of others. It guides us to act from our core rather than from an external set of rules and requirements. It exudes confidence without arrogance because what our inner knowing knows better than anything else is that we don't know everything. It has space for being wrong, for changing our minds, for taking a different direction. It has the capacity to sustain criticism in a way that urges growth. It has a willingness to question its own beliefs and those that are overlaid upon it from the outside world.

When we resolve our wounds and alchemize them into our weapons, we cease to be afraid to question ourselves. We unravel the threat of critique and feel safe with who we are. We no longer demand answers, perfection, or "right" behavior, and instead, we see each experience as an opportunity to deepen our inquiry and ultimately our understanding. Critical thought allows space for mistakes and reorientation; it is the bedrock of refinement. It trains us to have the capacity to hold multiple perspectives simultaneously: the essence of Yoga.

Despite our individual perceptions of the world, we can probably all agree that there is much turmoil in life, unless we are living in a willful state of denial or disassociation. As much as we desire to have a switch that can turn off difficulty, fear, and pain, if you've come this far in the book, you know it's not a realistic target. Instead, the practice of critical thinking empowers us to meet the turmoil in all its complexity—to show up fully in our moments of shame or anger, to open our ears to hear and our hearts to understand in moments when we struggle to allow other points of view. Critical thinking calls upon us to live Yoga in terms of reflection and resilience in order to help us to orient our experiences, both personal and collective, toward the juiciness of challenges. The ripples of change that result from a perspective shift can challenge what we previously trusted, causing us to grope in the dark for trustworthy ground or to turn inward to the foundation of our innate knowing.

With practice, we learn that trust oriented outside of ourselves is an invitation to question. With practice, we recognize that when we source trust from inside, we begin to scratch the surface of its existence, and we learn how to recognize it (or the absence of it) everywhere. Though many people carry difficult experiences that make trust hard to access, finding the opening to access trust that's sourced inside, independent of external circumstances or experiences, is how we begin to cultivate it. Inner trust can look like a complete redefinition of certain cultural norms. Yoga calls on us to redefine trust as an innate feeling rather than a blind faith in an external proof or authority. Inner trust requires the capacity to question many things, including our comforts, our accepted behaviors, our achievements, and our measurements of safety and success. Critical thought and self-trust are yoked together on the path of resilience. The experience of one is the access to the other, and both will result in resilience that is sustainable and mature. When we open up to this kind of trust, we encounter a way of living that is supportive to everyone, serving both the self and others, and we stretch the boundary of what is possible. Without denying our own needs or faults, we accept our truth and, in doing so, are able to extend our minds and hands beyond our limited perceptions to shape and form the world in which we desire to live.

Internal trust is the bedrock of building healthy boundaries and allows you to calibrate your compass arrow of guidance inwardly rather than outwardly. In doing this, we access true boundaries that keep us engaged with life rather than place limits on our possibilities or protect ourselves from further hurt. When we have a strong sense of our values and an orientation toward them, then we are able to push our limits. We feel less dependent upon defending or protecting ourselves and more anchored to our personal truth. This strength is a waypoint, not the destination, to external opinions or requests. It provides a pathway to engage without overextension and offers access to our fullest potential.

The Only Person That Knows What's Right for You Is You

Maybe it is a result of our education model that teaches us to stand quietly in a straight line, keep our hands to ourselves, do as we are told, or maybe it is a product of a professional environment that measures our successes on our ability to perform at the standards of others, or maybe it comes from our relationships that teach us that self-sacrifice is the highest form of care: regardless of where the idea originated, as a society, we are woefully dependent upon the feedback and acceptance of others to know our own truth. At this point, I hope this realization seems glaringly obvious. As long as we allow the external world to define our internal reality, we will be trapped in a cycle of fragility and dependency. When that is the case, we are miles away from sovereignty and autonomy and shrink from the idea of questioning what we have worked so hard to shape ourselves into in order to please others.

The painful truth is that the only person who can ever truly know you is you. I am the only person who will ever see the world through my eyes. I am the only person who will ever feel what I am feeling. My experience is unique to me, only me and forever. And no matter how much we try to fit into the preconceptions of others or the defined limitations that we are offered, we will only ever be able to be who we are. This terrifying truth is irrefutable, and we are the only ones who can discover it. With the application of critical thought, we can gingerly poke at the edges of our own identity. Who are we when no one defines who we are supposed to be? How do we show up when no one is looking? Who are we when everything we've been told, everything we've achieved, everything we've perfected is stripped away?

These perennial questions are the essence of Yoga and make up the deepest level of self-inquiry. They can break us apart if we dare to contemplate them, and they can set us free from our cages of definition and performance. The work of truly understanding ourselves allows us to take the load of expectation off the shoulders of others and put ourselves in the driver's seat of self-responsibility and autonomy. When we know who we are and what we value, we feel capable of making good choices for ourselves, choices that will also benefit our communities and our world. When we understand that our boundaries are not meant to keep others out but instead are the threads of remembering that keep us connected to who we really are, then we feel less inclined to use them to push others away and more willing to use them as the anchor points that open us up to bigger ideas, possibilities, and risks. Over time, this orientation to sovereignty of self creates the foundation needed to care for others (rather than take care of them), and the strength of our connections grows.

Practice and Application

Feel and Observe: Feel the feeling of trust inside. Where does it live in your body? Expand your awareness to the edge of who you are, to the boundary of your personal existence. How far can you expand? Breathe in and observe that you can fill up the space of your form with breath. Breathe and expand to the very edge of your being. Observe how the boundary feels. Observe how your boundary feels in your body. Is it small and tight? Is it large and fluid? Does it feel solid or permeable? Can you expand it?

Inquiry: What do you trust? How do you receive new information? Who are you when you are not trying to be something you are not?

Movement: Stand in a wide-legged stance. Begin with your hands joined at the center of your chest. As you inhale, extend both arms as far as you can reach out to either side (left and right) of the body. Keep breathing all the way out into your fingers. If possible, even hold the breath in for a moment, filling your entire form with breath. Exhale and return only your hands back to the center of your chest. Keep moving in this way for the next several cycles of the breath. Feel that with each arm extension you can expand the space that you are taking up a little more and a little more. Check in with your legs and feet to see whether they also need to widen and expand in order to adequately contain the full experience of your being filling up the boundaries of your skin. Linger in the fullness of form once you've completed the breath cycles.

Āsana and Energetics Suggestions:

Explore these āsanas *as a way to attenuate your knowledge, assimilating what is true for you and releasing what is not* (samāna/vyana).

CRP
Jaṭhara Parivartanāsana
Setu Bandha Sarvāṅgāsana
Paschimottānāsana
Śhavāsana

13

Metabolizing Our Hardships

True resilience requires tools to not only endure but to integrate our hardships as our lived experience. In addition to accountability and critical thought, alongside the importance of reflection and curiosity, we need ways to "suck the marrow" out of this life as well as to survive it. Survival alone isn't resilience, but when you join survival with joy, you are practicing the Yoga of your own wholeness, and this is a resilient life.

We must not only recognize but trust our own wholeness. When we move from trust in our choices and through our challenges, joy is a natural result. When trust is hard to find, joy is hard to find, and when trust is easy to find, joy is present in the tiniest places, in places where we never expected to find it. When we feel a sense of trust, joy effervesces up through our experiences. From years of practice, direct experience, and exhaustive experimentation, what I have observed is the more I can trust, the more joy I feel. And I began to wonder, if I can feel more joy, will I trust more deeply?

After a decade of exploration and processing, the experiment of joy and its relationship to trust has given way to a few key understandings about resilience and accessing the practice of Yoga.

The first discovery was that joy is not happiness. Sometimes joy results in happiness, but the two are not synonymous. According to the British publication *Psychologies* ("Joy vs Happiness," n.p.), joy is an emotion that is "consistent and cultivated internally," whereas happiness is an emotion that is felt in response to external experiences and is changeable as situations and experiences change.

Joy helps us to metabolize the pain and difficulty that we experience and the challenges that we face. Joy and the opportunity to allow pleasure to coexist with challenge grow our capacity for more challenge. In this way, joy is a bit like the digestive juices that break down our hardships and difficulties and make them assimilable. We can use joy to deconstruct our difficulties so that we can retain the nourishment from our experiences and release what doesn't serve us. When we are immersed in what feels unfamiliar, strange, and scary and yet still find beauty, we are in the process of assimilating our experiences. Whether it is in the moment of occurrence or in the spaces of reflection, the recognition of beauty and vitality even in the most difficult of places is essential to our resilience.

The second realization was that finding beauty does not negate suffering. This idea that it does is perhaps the biggest fallacy relevant to resilience. When we begin to unhook our need to keep beauty and pain separate, we move into Yoga. Joy and beauty can and do exist simultaneously and perpetually alongside our challenges and pain, and when we work to yoke or harness them together rather than separate or categorize them, we are in the practice and experience of Yoga. When times are hard, owning and accessing our experiences of joy can feel like a betrayal of the difficulty. So, we create (or have been taught) strategies to avoid feeling the full scope of our experiences. We work to deny beauty when there is suffering because we need to appropriately acknowledge the pain and because our suffering justifies our wariness and reinforces our belief that trust is in short supply. It's hard to feel joy when we are feeling pain but not impossible, because joy exists within and in concert with all our external circumstances.

Negativity Bias

When times are hard, we are wired to withdraw and protect ourselves. When we are faced with a challenge, we are programmed to assume the worst so that we are compelled to survive. This is called "negativity bias." In his book, *Hardwiring Happiness*, Dr. Rick Hanson explores the fact that our brains are wired toward negativity in support of survival. We log and categorize these experiences so that we can stay safe in the future. In addition, when we have a negative experience, it imprints almost instantly into our memory. We barely have a moment to assess the situation before our brains have recorded it. Then, we move forward holding on to the feeling, resonance, and tone of the threat, regardless of the larger context of the situation. For example, if we were at a surprise party having a wonderful time, and for five minutes we choked on our birthday cake, the brain would remember the life-threatening experience more clearly and more readily than the hours of joy that preceded and followed it. The memory of that survival challenge would imprint instantly and color all our future experiences with birthday cake and perhaps even surprise parties.

Negativity bias colors our lived experience. It turns our attention to our context and overwrites the content that is always present. It makes our memories of past experiences paramount and leaves very little room for new possibilities. It assumes the worst as a means of protection, often from threats that do not exist beyond the scope of our mind. Negativity bias impedes joy because it tunes our perspective to the "bad" or dangerous possibilities in every situation. Our instrument of perception seeks out opportunities for harm, often bypassing the "good" and beautiful that is right in front of us. Negativity bias pushes us to look for snakes in the flower bed rather than smell the flowers. It shields us from the nurturing qualities of joy, beauty, and wonder. It prevents us from receiving the emotional sustenance we need to metabolize our experiences of hardship and instead makes us hyper vigilant to more difficulty. Luckily, negativity bias can be countered and retrained, but it takes work.

To imprint positive experiences into our memory, our thoughts, and our emotions, we have to pay attention to and work at recalibrating our perception to what is present from moment to moment rather than reinforcing our past experiences. Recalibration requires that we challenge the idea that we are fully formed and defined by our past difficulties and traumas and that we invest a great deal of attention, effort, and willingness to unhook ourselves from our ideas of threat and insecurity. I have a friend who calls this "radical affirmation," and she practices it every day. Though she has experienced many hardships in her life, she tunes herself to see the beauty available in each moment, and she admits that sometimes it's easier than others. When I'm in a bad mood, my friend's commitment to excavating the beauty feels frustrating—"Why can't she just get on board with the fact that having a flat tire is awful?! And stop telling me about how beautiful the view is from the side of the road?!" To be clear, radical affirmation isn't a bypass of what is real; it is an addition to it. My friend never denies the hardships of the moment. She simply adds to them with her observations of the beauty that also exists, affirming that there is always a bigger picture available to see. Because beauty is perpetually present even in the most devastating situations, it is up to the viewer to notice it. Our awareness is key in overcoming the reinforcement of our negativity bias, but it does not require a denial of what is. Committing to noticing the beauty amidst the often painful and ugly reality is an intense practice, and it's not for the faint of heart. What it is, though, is a doorway to greater resilience, joy, and potential.

The third recognition about joy emphasizes that we need positive experiences to create an internal storehouse of joy reference points, but it's not easy. Because negative experiences imprint immediately while positive experiences require time and attention to make a mark on our psyche, it takes greater commitment to build our joy reserves. For example, if we pass through 12 traffic lights and 11 of them are green but the last one is red, we are more likely to remember the one red light than the previous 11 green ones. The protective survival strategy that works to guard us from threat is difficult to counter. The same reason that we are not wired to remember the green lights is also why we are not wired to remember the flowers in the spring, and if we are to rewire for positivity, we have to work at it. The unexpected and celebratory feelings that bubble up every time the blooms return after a long, cold winter are exciting precisely because we're not structured to hold that memory. We are designed to dread the season of cold and dark and to prepare ourselves so that we can survive it. But our brains do not yearn to celebrate the spring, and instead the new season is something that may catch us by surprise. Some of us may have to work at finding the joy in it, which could be easily missed if we aren't paying attention.

Joy Takes Work

Additionally, to understand the importance of joy, we must recognize that emotion is generative. Yoga teaches us that our feelings generate more of themselves. When we feel afraid, the feeling of fear itself generates more fear. When we feel doubtful, there is more doubt to feel. Fortunately, when we feel and experience joy, it also generates more joy. Yet, because joy is harder to focus on than its opposite, we often miss the opportunity to generate it in our lives. It is imperative in this modern age, in which a joy infusion is necessary to metabolize our hardships, that we begin to make the effort. We have so many challenges and difficulties. Around every corner, we seem to have the opportunity to be afraid, to doubt, and to be terrifyingly uncertain, making the work of metabolizing our suffering a necessity for resilience. Recall the last time you had to take a test. When you doubted that you could pass that test, it increased the doubt, consequently generating more doubt and more doubt and more doubt. Maybe it woke you up in the middle of the night, afraid that you were going to fail the test. Maybe you wake up even now, years later, from the residual fear that lingers from that long-past experience. Because our difficulties imprint so quickly and deeply in our bodies and minds, countering those effects takes hard work and diligence. In order to imprint positive experiences on the psyche, we must linger in them longer, absorb more of their detail and nuance, and recall them more often. Positive reflection requires more time, more attention, more effort, and more will.

Emotion and feeling are generative, and if we're not committing as much time to generating a reserve of joy as we do habitually generating negativity, then we find ourselves in places where it's difficult to see beyond our challenges and hardships. When that threshold is reached, it becomes harder and harder to digest and metabolize our difficulties when they inevitably arise. We experience feelings that have culturally defined labels, like overwhelm, anxiety, frustration, sensitivity. We can feel helpless and hopeless. We experience despair and depression. And we forget that these feelings are only one dimension of the multi-dimensional life that we have an opportunity to live. It's precisely these experiences that need an infusion of joy. The opportunities for joy that present themselves may be small and hidden and require work to access, but they are there, if we dare to look. Whether that work is intense or easy varies based on the opportunity and advantage available, but let's be clear: it is always work. The cultivation of our capacity to experience more and to pay attention to the details that can open us to joy is hard work, and it's completely up to each of us individually to put forth the effort. Joy is something that, if we dare to open ourselves to access and experience it, is everywhere and accessible more often than we realize. Though it may be approached and felt differently for me than for you, the opportunity to feel it, experience it, and see it is literally everywhere. Walking through the woods on a rainy day brings me joy, digging fingers into dark soil brings my friend joy, dancing until they drop brings yet another friend joy. It could be cool water on a hot day or warm, cozy blankets and a crackling fire in the cold of winter. All these things coexist with our challenges, yet they can fill us up. Every one of us could open our front door and see something joyful if we try, because the essence of life itself is miraculous, according to Yoga. But we must train our eyes to see it, our ears to attune to it, our bodies to soften and receive it.

> Whoever you are, no matter how lonely,
> the world offers itself to your imagination ... [Oliver, *New and Selected Poems*, p. 110].

When we emerged into this life, everyone agreed that our mere existence was a miracle. Those in attendance "oohed" and "aahed" over our tiny ten fingers and tiny ten toes; even our cries brought joy to the room. And the truth is we are a miracle: an incredibly complex and elaborate combination of history, biology, time, lineage, and culture. Whatever our past, whatever our history, wherever we come from, everybody thought, in the moment of our first emergence, that we were a miracle. My question is simple: When did that stop? When did we become so bound to the identification with our pain and hardship that we forgot our very existence was miraculous? Regardless of the reason, once it's begun, the forgetting grows, it consumes, and it hungers, until it starves us of our connection to the vitality that is always all around us unless we work to keep it in check. The reality of our existence is simple: we've never stopped being miraculous. Though we might have forgotten, we continue to be a living miracle. Though the act of remembering our miraculous existence might be hard work, it is work whose worth far exceeds the effort.

Negativity bias and the teachings of Yoga tell us that we are wired to forget, but they also instruct us that it's our privilege to remember. Concealing our memory is part of the dance of divinity, not because of cruelty or for punishment, but because the opportunity to remember is so joyful. So, when we remember that we were once a miracle, we can begin to remember that the piece of us that is miraculous has never left. Though we may have forgotten it, though it may be hidden from us, we have the capacity to remember. And in the simple act of remembering, every minuscule detail of our existence is an opportunity for joy. When we can become mesmerized by the tiniest pebble on the ground or the dandelion growing through the crack in the sidewalk, our awe can be overwhelmingly joyful. When we lose ourselves in a reverie of wonder when listening to the chorus of our favorite song or are overcome by our lover's gaze, we are being invited into the heart of joy. Since we all have the capacity to remember that we're a miracle, eventually we can reach a tipping point where we no longer feel unable to remember. Even if we don't always do it, we know that we are capable of remembering that everything, even the challenges that help us grow and build our capacity and make us suffer, has a miraculous quality to it. All of this can happen more and more often simply by choosing to turn our vision in the direction of the miracle.

Joy as a Practice

Joy is a practice and not an easy one. Even though we are a miracle, and we emerged into this miraculous space, the experience and cultivation of joy requires attention, commitment, and discipline. Because we carry the weight of our memories, impressions, challenges, difficulties, and lessons, the load we carry can start to feel heavy after a while. And the heavier the load, the easier the forgetting. Some of our loads are much weightier than others, and some of our loads are so heavy that even the thought of trying to access joy feels like just another rock we must haul in our backpack. Yet, when we experience joy and take the time to access it, we may notice that it lightens our load. It takes off some of the weight, the heaviness of our existence, and it gives us access to more lightness and possibility. Yoga and resilience are practices of "more." The point is not to attempt to transcend what is nor is it to move in a linear direction toward an outcome or achievement that is insistent on disregarding our inner experience. Rather, it is an invitation to fully engage with whatever and wherever we find ourselves and recognize that every moment of engagement holds within it the opportunity for more engagement, for more experience, for more moments. In this way, even our mess is joyful, sacred, holy.

Yoga as resilience is a practice that builds rather than reduces. It teaches us that we're way more alike than we are different. We're way more connected than we are separate. We're way more together than we are apart. Unfortunately, this idea is often reduced to some sort of notion of unification, but in truth, it's much bigger than that. It is inclusion: a recognition that all the parts make up the whole. Yoga says we are all yoked together, tied together into one big knot. All the individuals make up *the everything*. When we realize, through that daring act of thinking and questioning, that we're all connected, then it makes us more responsible and more thoughtful about how we choose to act. It gives us access to more joy and more curiosity. It opens us up to more resilience.

Though we have been trained to only experience joy once we have achieved the necessary successes, it's a fallacy that we must earn our right to be joyful. Based on our education and early instruction, many of us have cultivated lives based on chasing successes with the promise that someday we can land in the space of joy. Then, we spend years not seeing what's right in front of us, not remembering that we and everyone else have been and will always be a miracle. When we stop subscribing to the learned belief system of the dominant culture of North America and begin to apply our own critical analysis to what is "real," we start practicing seeing things differently. A shifting perspective can open up possibilities that don't require us to achieve anything to be worthy of experiencing everything. When we are liberated from the ideas that everything, including ourselves, must be perfectly correct or that we must do everything right, we remember that we don't have to make money or please people or look this way or act that way in order for more to be accessible. It's literally always here. Yet, the challenge remains. Though it perpetually exists, we often don't see it, and it doesn't fall into neat and clean categories of delineation. The difficulty is that the "more" that Yoga gives us access to isn't just the "good." It's also everything else, and we don't like that. Instead, we mount a resistance against the more by choosing to focus only on the good. When we don't feel or attain what we define as good or right, we have a tendency to feel as if we've been betrayed. We weave a story that goodness doesn't exist for us in order to justify our blindness or shield our pain. We create the belief that joy is only for other people. Perhaps it is this very thought that joy is inaccessible that provides the opportunity and pushes us to find it in our lives. In some strange and mysterious way, we paradoxically find joy most often from its opposite. When we experience the depths of despair, we become aware that the heights of joy are truly accessible. This process is often a brutal one and requires willpower and determination (*icchā shakti*), awareness (*Chit shakti*), and courage (*vira bhava*).

The challenge of making the picture whole is not to be underestimated. It is much easier to reduce our understanding to only what we can see and to assume that is all that ever will be. Plus, how we gauge the level of our life challenges is based on the scale of measurement that we have learned rather than felt or explored. This scale is often measured dichotomously, placing what is good in opposition to what is bad and demanding that we exhaustively strive for the good because we've been told that it's a failure to feel bad. What if we entertain the idea that feeling only good and right is wrong? What if what we are striving to accomplish is incorrect and actually exacerbating the problem we are trying to correct? Do we dare have the courage to think critically about it? Can we bravely ponder the theory that we are built from such power and such beauty and such potential and such possibility, that we are so miraculous that we actually have access, capacity, ability, strength, to feel *both* good and bad? Can we consider that perhaps feeling bad and all of the nuances of feeling and challenge are just as rich in some ways as feeling good? When we recognize that we're designed to feel both, we open up the possibility of having full access to it all. This awareness frees us from the necessity of having to slice off parts of ourselves or cut off other things, people, or experiences that fall into the negative category. The result is that we don't have to eliminate the negative in order to experience joy. We don't have to wait. It's accessible to us now. Even in the hardest of times.

13. *Metabolizing Our Hardships*

> Every human being is an unprecedented miracle. One tries to treat them as the miracles they are, while trying to protect oneself against the disasters they've become [No Name, p. 10].
>
> —James Baldwin

Spiritual Bypassing

The allowance for the whole picture to exist is a direct remedy to the modern attachment to spiritual bypassing. Spiritual bypassing, according to psychotherapist John Welwood, is "using spiritual ideas and practices to sidestep personal, emotional 'unfinished business,' to shore up a shaky sense of self, or to belittle basic needs, feelings, and developmental tasks, all in the name of enlightenment" (*Toward a Psychology of Awakening*, p. 207).

Often spiritual bypassing is expressed, but not always, as a desire to make everything love, light, and goodness all the time. It can and often does deny the full spectrum of our or others' lived experiences and cuts us off from so much of the energy and vitality that's available to us as living beings. In recognizing that this process actively denies the vast scope of our lived experience, is it possible that the refusal to experience joy is also spiritual bypassing?

In our modern world, there seems to be great importance placed on taking a stance on feeling, either refusing to feel excited, happy, joyful or refusing to acknowledge pain, suffering, and difficulty. Is the refusal to allow ourselves to feel joy or to celebrate keeping us bound to a sense of importance or of self-preservation? Do we need to deny that everything has its own miraculous existence in order to justify or validate our own discomforts or challenges? It's surprising how often the outright refusal to make space for joy and beauty has become commonplace. It's easy to theoretically acknowledge the many miracles of existence, including but not limited to ourselves, but because we have such a strong resistance to being wrong, we often do not allow ourselves to yield to it. We have so much fear that we will be duped by celebrating something that might turn out to be not what we thought. We abhor the possibility of being taken advantage of or being gullible. We prefer to know without ever having the experiences that earn the knowing.

We have a resistance to affirming the miraculous nature of life not because it's not miraculous but because we don't trust ourselves. The denial of joy is how we can bypass our opportunity to feel the full capacity of what is available to us in our lives. If we notice that we go down a road of challenge or difficulty or despair, and somehow that road seems to go on forever, it might indicate that we are cultivating resistance to the critical thought that would show us that the endless road could be partially our choice. Take, for example, an unhealthy relationship that seems impossible to get out of, though friends and family have urged the change, offered support, listened with care. In feeling that we are unable to leave, we are almost always overlooking the truth that we made the choice to stay over and over again, resulting in the deepening of our pain even as we desperately want to escape it.

Because emotion is generative, we can apply our awareness and discernment to choose what we want to cultivate. With the tools of critical thought, awareness, and discernment, we can generate the recognition of our desire without having to deny the reality of how we feel. We begin to build capacity to hold multifarious experiences and truths at once, and in doing so, we step into Yoga and begin to become buoyant with our resilience. This pivot of perspective can have a far-reaching impact too. When we apply discernment and choice to our emotions, we are modeling this behavior for others, perhaps even inspiring them to replicate the process. So, when one thousand of us, or ten thousand of us, or one hundred thousand of us, or a million of us refuse to let joy in because we don't want to be duped or proven wrong, then that refusal multiplies.

Not allowing ourselves the opportunity to be wrong robs us of the opportunity to learn, to grow, and to celebrate the moments as they are. When everything comes under scrutiny, we can't immerse ourselves in the experience of the moment because we could be "wrong" about it. This approach generates self-doubt and the absence of trust. Instead, we could choose to celebrate regardless of the possibility of being wrong. How many times have we started a new relationship with a partner and said despite the depth and intensity of our feelings, "I don't really know if this is love or not; maybe I'm wrong"? The result is that we won't take the risk. Because we are afraid of being foolish or because we cannot guarantee the security of it lasting forever, we won't let ourselves fully love. We choose not to generate love and instead compound our fear, distrust, and separation. Our choice is shaping our experience, sometimes consciously and sometimes unconsciously, and robbing us of the opportunity to feel joy, to metabolize the very fears and doubts that are creating the challenge.

Can we shift our cultural idea of not wanting to be wrong and, in doing so, respond to our lives in a way that metabolizes our difficulties?

Can we celebrate everything that feels awe-striking and allow ourselves to feel joy in the uncomplicated things? Can we dare to experience joy in the tiniest and most insignificant of places, even if it doesn't last or it proves us wrong? I struggle to find the negative outcome of allowing ourselves to experience joy. In addition, when we can hold to the idea that being wrong is not negative, we can begin to grow our capacity to experience the full spectrum of life.

I was a super nerd in school, not with every class but with the ones that mattered. I can't remember any of the correct answers from all the tests for which I studied so hard. Yet, I can still remember what I did wrong. Learning from what we get right or from our achievements and our perfections isn't a requirement, but we necessarily learn from getting things wrong and by reflecting on our failures and our imperfections. Learning alone is something that can be celebrated rather than avoided, and that may be the point. How would it shift the measure of our days if there was room to fail, to fall down, to make mistakes? Would joy be more accessible if we allowed its opposite to also be present? From each experience of joy, and the companion experiences of surrender and acceptance, we find that the hardships we face might not be as unbearable as we imagined. Our mistakes won't suffocate us or annihilate us nor cut us off from what's available in this life. They can become the fertile ground of our joy.

What do you celebrate? There is a nuance between what we're grateful for and what we celebrate. Sometimes we celebrate things and become grateful for them, and other times we are grateful for things and then learn how to celebrate them. The two expressions of joy are not mutually exclusive nor indivisibly bound. But when we access joy to help us metabolize our difficulties, gratitude and celebration can be a starting point and the result. So, let's consider what we celebrate. What kind of requirements do we put around what we are grateful for? What demands and expectations do we impose upon our rejoicing? Are they part of the resistance to joy? Can we dare to challenge the need for perfection even in our joy? Do we require the most beautiful sunset for it to be worth celebrating or could it be mediocre? Can we appreciate the fact that particulates in the air, i.e., air pollution, create the most stellar sunsets and choose to celebrate it not in spite of that fact but in unison with it? This is the Yoga of joy, and this is the path of resilience, the path of allowing it *all* to coexist. Then the practice is noticing the opportunities to be grateful for more than you thought you could be. Loosen the restrictions on what is worthy of celebrating, and see how the joy floods in.

Tools for Joy

Curiosity

Recognize that we don't know everything. Maybe we don't even know a fraction of anything. Curiosity places our hearts into the hands of the mystery and gives space to not have it all figured out. When we become curious, we become more aware that we are perceiving less than a fraction of what's available to us. That invites us to breathe a little. When what we trust or what we deem to be true or right is in reality only ever a fraction of the whole, we will never know enough. So instead, we can choose to surrender to the not knowing and get curious about everything. Then, everything becomes a discovery. Everything becomes an opportunity to be awed. Even the pain becomes an opportunity to discover more sensation, more dimension, more texture, more depth. Even fear becomes a place to explore as opposed to a place to eliminate.

Since elimination is the beginning of the well-worn trail of forgetting, we can recognize that tendency and bring our awareness and curiosity to it. Eventually, we may not want to forget anymore. We won't want to turn a blind eye to everything that is now evident or sweep it under the rug. In this approach to joy, we don't have to pretend like the trouble never existed or go back to the way things were. Joy is the vehicle for living forward, and curiosity is its captain. In opening up to joy, we can be awed, amazed, shocked, and heartbroken. But whatever we are, we will be more. Because that is what life is. An opportunity for "more" is available no matter what life we're living.

Curiosity is a tool to invoke joy. And joy is a tool to digest our pain. And none of these experiences make any of the rest go away. So, dare to wonder what draws us in? What magnetizes us? It doesn't have to be on the spectrum of positivity to be inspiring. What is intriguing? That's where to start. If you are drawn in, go towards it. Seek out the miraculous in it. Know that everything, all things are a source of joy. In addition, become aware of what you are attracted to and what generates aversions. Take care to avoid cultivating attachments to what you don't want. We can become curious about the things that we don't want to see and begin to wonder why we don't want to acknowledge the miracle in those places too. Take the chance to be curious, and see what joy emerges from the risk. Utilizing joy as the catalyst to metabolize pain and suffering anchors us to resilience. It invites us to enter into the experience of Yoga and pivot our perspective toward more.

Risk

Take a chance. Do something differently. Take the long way home, try a new food, dance on the street corner, laugh from your belly. Dare to embarrass yourself. Trust in the innocence of your heart to guide you into beauty and awe. Sing out loud. Don't worry so much about being liked and discover the joy of liking yourself no matter what anyone else thinks. Say "yes" to life. Sure, bring your lessons, your cautions, your fears, and say "yes" anyway. Do the thing that your soul longs for but your mind calls ridiculous. Be ridiculous. Take the risk to experience, even if there is no guarantee of success. Dare to fail; dare to fall. Jump anyway. If the music moves you, take the risk to dance, regardless of who's watching. Laugh louder than appropriate. Do the thing that your mind is wrestling with. Step a toe over the line and see what happens. Potential lies inside the desire you feel, and possibility is what unfolds when you take the risk to pursue it.

Love

In the words of Mary Oliver, "let the soft animal of your body love what it loves" (New and Selected Poems, p. 110). Don't just like things; don't just approve. Give even the simple things all that you've got. Love the flavor of a strawberry, love the colors of the sky, love the sound of water trickling on your windowsill, love with abandon that which you love. Don't hesitate and resist the urge to envelop your friend in your arms. Move toward that which draws you in. Open your heart to the lessons it will teach you, even if the lesson feels like heartbreak. There are some things you can only know from the inside. Like Yoga and resilience, love is a practice and an experience. Seek out both of them. Be washed in love. Open your eyes to the sky and the grass and feel love emanating from them. Even when the experience of relational love seems far away, find your communion with what is close. Love the way the wind blows; love the shafts of light across your kitchen table. Love the bird song in the spring. Let it take your breath away and make your pulse quicken. Love the life you are in and watch it generate more.

Laughter

Laugh a lot and at every opportunity. Laugh at yourself. Laugh at the joke that isn't funny. Laugh with others often. Laugh even when you aren't sure you feel like it. Laugh out loud. Guffaw, snort, or chuckle. Giggle softly. Fake it. Pretend to laugh and watch how it evolves into unstoppable roars. Watch a funny movie; listen to your favorite comedian. Tell a joke. Fall down in the mud and howl. Though it is cliché, it is also true: laughter is the best medicine. Do it often and with friends. Take Action. Don't wait for joy to fall into your lap. Seek it.

Silence

Power down. Dare to be free of distraction and busyness. Joy is not the outcome of some great success or achievement. It's not the ability to juggle all challenges with grace. Joy is the hum of contentment ("*santosha*" in Sanskrit) that is perpetually vibrating under the surface of our lives. We must get quiet to hear it. Very quiet. We must learn to listen into the silence, into and through the cacophony of thoughts, worries, and demands until we arrive at the space within ourselves that is untouched, unaffected, unstruck by the play of our identity or the pull of the world. The Yogis call this "*pratyahara*" in Sanskrit, meaning withdrawal of the senses. Only this can provide the necessary space to remember the self beneath and within all the external distractions.

Solitude

Be alone. Silence is enhanced by aloneness. Sustain your initial period of loneliness and disconnection long enough to come through to your aloneness. Solitude is a necessary tool for experiencing joy, even for those who feel terrified of it. The experience of joy requires us to be in harmony with ourselves. To be tuned in to the inner gift of our "one wild and precious life" (Oliver, New and Selected Poems, p. 94) creates an opportunity to access joy without the requirement of external alignment. When we remember that our individual life is a gift, even in its most challenging moments, even amidst extreme hardship, even when our environment isn't providing or reflecting that gift, then we are dancing cheek to cheek with joy. This level of realization is available primarily when we strip away all outside influences, striving, and distractions (even the ones that "make us happy") and dare to spend some time with and in the gift of our lives.

Beauty

Whether getting lost in a work of art, a natural landscape, or your lover's eyes, immerse yourself in beauty. Dare to see the beautiful aspects of even the atrocious things. Victor Frankl emerged from the most horrific experience of survival in a Nazi concentration camp with an appreciation for the tiny and almost invisible beauties of the world. Try looking where you least expect it and see whether you can find something lovely. Start close in, as Whyte reminds us, and sink in. Expand your vocabulary to include words that describe the beautiful. Use those words often. Read poetry. Walk barefoot in the dew-covered grass. Be awed by the simple and enraptured by the complex. Don't take the little things for granted. Open your vision fully to take in even the beautiful aspects of the most mundane occurrences.

Gratitude

In "The Work That Reconnects," based on the teachings developed by author, environmentalist, and spiritual teacher Joanna Macy, participants are taught a "spiral" journey through the stages of difficulty and reconnection (Work That Reconnects Network, n.p.). One of the most important and potent tools of this spiral is the work of gratitude. Gratitude is the gateway to appreciating the beauty that surrounds you, the spaces that you occupy, the history that shores you up, and the opportunities that lie ahead. Gratitude is an action, a salve, and a resting place. It softens the sharp edges of our experiences and welcomes new perspectives. Gratitude is courageous. It dares to find ways to open up to where we are (regardless of its imperfections) and to hold pain in concert with beauty, tears alongside laughter, and loss together with love. Gratitude does not presuppose a gain nor wane in the face of loss. It is available in every situation, and it is up to us to access it. Gratitude is a necessary skill of resilience and the natural result that unfolds with Yoga. It is a powerful threshold to understanding the bigger picture and invites agency.

The tools to access joy are not exclusive nor are they only available to the most privileged few. They are everywhere, they are timeless, and they are here for anyone who chooses to access them. They don't demand grand gestures or seismic shifts of opinion. They don't demand that we disregard our pain or deny the reality we are in. What they do is create space in our experiences of collapse and constriction. They widen the lens to allow for a larger and more benevolent depiction to be braided into the story alongside the difficulty. They help us to digest our difficulties and integrate our hardships. But most importantly, they are always available. They are piano players in bomb raids, dances in the downpours, they are reconciliations of regrets, and wordless smiles to strangers. They are often simple and unspoken yet profoundly impactful. They stretch meaning to include the fullness of our lives and uncover the forgotten details of the miracles we all are. The tools for joy are direct access points to resilience and are the true experience of a Yogic life. They require practice, will, determination, and diligence for the entirety of our short and precious time.

Practice and Application

Feel and Observe: Recall a joyful experience. Reach as far back in your memories as necessary to access a moment of feeling joy. Then, as if looking at a snapshot of that moment, allow yourself to sink into it. See the expression on your own face. Feel the energy of the space surrounding this moment captured in time. Observe the sensations that are present in your body. Feel the quality and texture of your breath. Slowly observe the details of the moment fading away but allow the feeling of joy to remain. Feel this feeling expand into the space where the story once was. Take a few moments to observe and open up to the feeling of joy pulsing within you, free of conditions or expectations.

Inquiry: In what ways do you welcome joy into your life? In what ways do you block it?

Movement: Dance!! Skip!! Do cartwheels!!

Āsana and Energetics Suggestions:

Explore these āsanas as a gateway to expansion, joy, enthusiasm, and integration (udāna/vyāna).

Bālāsana
Adho Mukha Śhvānāsana
Vīrabhadrāsana II
Prasārita Pādottānāsana
Trikonāsana
Śhalabhāsana
Sphinx
Setu Bandha Sarvāṅgāsana
Śhavāsana

14

Resiliency Is Maturity

Living a resilient life might be easier than you think. In fact, you might be living resiliently right now, engaging in and from a space of Yoga but never identifying it as anything special or important. Because that is precisely what living resiliently is all about: living life as it is without trying to spotlight the adversities that we have overcome and without demanding things to be different because we deserve it. Resilience is the recognition that we are meeting life rather than requiring life to meet us. This way of thinking, responding, and moving in the world is one that resonates maturity and responsibility, and age is not the determinant.

To be mature means to reach "an advanced stage of mental or emotional development"; to be "careful and thorough" (Lexico, "Mature," n.p.). The etymology of the word points to a ripening and readiness. Maturation, though supported by the experience gleaned over the years, is irrespective of age and is the key to resilience. When we ripen, we coalesce our lessons into a developed and integrated knowing. We have digested our past pains and traumas and choose to draw upon their lessons in our lived experience. We recognize both the sweetness and the difficulty of where we've been, where we are now, and where we are going without diminishing the mysterious and unknown nature of our experiences. Maturity expresses itself as a recognition of a long timeline, one of which we are just a character in a larger story, not the star. Maturity allows space for the unknown and simultaneously stays curious and critical rather than complacent and apathetic. Maturity lends a quiet and persistent engagement to the complexity and shies away from oversimplification and reduction.

When we have risked everything to question and explore the nature of our experiences and emerged from the underworld of self-recognition into the realization that we are a part of a much bigger experience, then we begin to approach our present and future experiences with these tools and understandings in tow. Because we have dared to question ourselves, questioning the world no longer feels as threatening as it did during our formation. We more readily drop the expectations and requirements of outcome and instead relish each experience for the opportunity for development, deepening, comprehension, and awe. Life shifts from the arc of achievement into the spiral of exploration and experimentation and ultimately becomes more enjoyable to live.

Please don't confuse enjoyment with ease. As we gain resilience, life does not become easier to live, but it does become juicier, fuller of flavor and dimension. Maturity shifts our focus from plot development to character development. We no longer strive to simply chart our course of success by marking what we can do or the achievements we collect and shift instead into the experience of being what we are, whatever that is, wherever it happens. We become interested in developing the character of the self that we have the opportunity to discover and cultivate. Maturity invites us to see that our biggest contributions aren't material in nature and that material things won't fix anyone or anything. When we are responding from a mature place, we are stepping into sovereignty where we become accountable for our role in each interaction and aware that our responses are shaping the story in which we are living in the very moment that we are living it.

With maturity, we learn how to hold our feelings, bring awareness to our patterns, and be fiercely compassionate to ourselves and others. There is room for faults, improvements, and constant change, though rarely is there room for perfection. The space engenders an internal sense of freedom, referred to as "*moksha*" in Sanskrit. Not to be confused with happiness, freedom is allowing, accepting, and sometimes brutal. Often referred to as "*Vairāgya*," or "detachment" (or non-attachment as mentioned previously), this freedom has space for all possibilities to coexist. Though we may continue to strive to be in alignment with all that we've discovered, we feel less concerned about the outcomes. We grant ourselves permission to slow down and allow the moments to shape us, and we dare to do so. As one of my most revered teachers, Bayo Akomolafe, says often and in repetition, "Times are urgent, we must slow down." Slowing down is required for knowing, knowing ourselves with all of our shadows and our illuminations, knowing the world around us and our relationship with it, knowing others to the point that we have seen ourselves in their eyes. When we slow down, we bring with us the possibility of taking in more, of having space for complexity, but when we react and enact old familiar patterns or simply do what we've been told, we miss the opportunities to make our moments our education, to make our troubles the friction that shapes us and ultimately shapes our world.

132

Maturity Is Holding Complexity

We would likely all agree that the world is a complex place. Some would say it is more complex now than ever. We feel overwhelmed, we scramble to make sense of destruction, to understand the widening divides, and for many, to find simple and peaceful answers to the eruption of problems. Yet, we continually fall short of discovering what we seek. Our demands for understanding from others don't offer solutions, and our intense devotion to simplicity leaves us disappointed and dejected as the problems mount and grow. Though we understand that the world is theoretically complex and impossible to fully comprehend, we continue to demand that it be reduced to manageable parts and, knowingly or not, contribute to turning the complexity into complication. Maturity provides the space needed to hold and honor the complexity and helps to minimize the complications that arise from the personal resistance and reaction born from immaturity. When we are able to hold the complexity of any given experience without the demand for its reduction or elimination, we create space for more rather than less.

Lessening and managing the whole is often expressed as the impetus to control, reduce, and diminish. When we feel overwhelmed by the "more," we crave the experience of less. We long to decrease the intricacy, to mitigate the multitudes, and to contract or hide from the differences. Our desire to limit the fullness of our experiences and relationships to only what we feel we can manage is our evidence of underdeveloped or misappropriated trust, belief, identity, and attachment. In maturity, we no longer seek to abridge our moments. We source our steadiness from within, regardless of the tumult of outer circumstance. We make choices on how, when, and whether to respond from that steadiness that has weathered storms in the past and feel able, even willing, to step into the torrents again, to take in more. However, more means more. When we strive to have a direct experience of this agreed upon complexity rather than reducing it to something more manageable, we step into *more* and all that it brings. More life, more joy, more complexity, more complication, more frustration, more. And in a resilient life, we grow our capacity to hold more and all the complexity that comes with it. This is precisely the experience of Yoga.

We can play with the idea of holding more complexity by thinking about perspective and its relationship to truth and facts. Every person on the planet "sees" from a very individual perspective ("*sva*" in Sanskrit). A way of "seeing," experiencing, feeling is unique to each individual. Yes, there is overlap based on shared history, culture, and experience, but even these aspects of perspective can ever and only be perceived individually by the one perceiving. I don't mean this to sound too complex, so here's an example: I am at the market buying apples. Based on a host of factors, including what I've been taught a good apple looks like, feels like, and smells like, as well as what I've learned about the place and growing conditions of that apple, I determine which apples are best to purchase, and I put them in my bag. A dozen other people come to the apple bin and go through a similar process of choice, but each one aligns their choice with their own unique set of variables based on their individual experiences. This process could have all of us agreeing on what is a good apple, completely disagreeing about it, or landing somewhere amidst the innumerable assessments in between, but the understanding that underlies all our arguments is unique and exclusively our own.

It's fascinating, really, how truly diverse—defined as "showing a great deal of variety; very different" (Lexico, "Diverse," n.p.)—our perspectives are on the same concrete things. As a species, we are infinitely unique and complex. We are a living, breathing expression of more. Yet, rather than recognize the beauty in this, we often desire to get everyone to see the world through our eyes, something that they can't nor will ever be able to do. We use arguments, pleas, admonishment, and insults. We use coercion, manipulation, demand, and "proof." We pull out all the stops to bring the "other" into our way of seeing the world rather than make room for the complexity of perspective. Maturity recognizes that holding space for all perspectives at once is also a choice. And when we hold more rather than reduce to less, we are practicing the highly refined skill of resilience. Resilience equates with making space for a variety of opinions and ideas, allowing us to "see" things differently without making one perspective wrong and another right. And perhaps the most quintessentially Yogic concept when dealing with complexity is the agreement to engage with the contradictions that emerge by permitting these contradictions to coexist. When we recognize that our way of seeing the world is simply one out of eight billion possible perspectives, we become more flexible and receptive to the vast scope of unique perspectives. We expand our capacity to hold more.

Now, if we can lean into the possibility that no one views the world in exactly the same way, we can begin to loosen the grip on the *need* for everyone to see it one way. We can begin to stretch the edges of our own personal perception to allow for more: more questions, more curiosities, more contradictions, and more doubt and frustration too. We can stop trying to get everyone on the same page, and instead increase the size of the book. We can open to *more* and watch with interest our tendencies to simplify as a means to evade the discomforts of a widening horizon. Maybe we can even challenge our own fixed ideas in a way that opens us up to more possibility, more creativity, more understanding, more lessons, and more maturity.

Rather than shielding and sheltering our highly sensitive natures (that "feel" the world around us), we can begin to see our sensitivity as a superpower that everyone has in varying degrees. We can recognize the threshold of opening that expands our understanding, and we can choose to open up to it, to take in the lessons it offers (even if it doesn't align with what we want). In mature experience, we transform our triggers into the tools that we use skillfully, not to change others or demand moderation in order to alleviate our discomforts, but instead to broaden our perspectives and increase our own capacity. This Yoga invites us to move through the world as a dance of differing perspectives, yielding, swaying, and meeting each one as a part of the whole. The intensity of the rhythm is dictated only by our willingness to hear, wonder, meet, and receive.

Maturity doesn't "fix" anything. It might not make anyone feel more comfortable, most especially *you*, but it might make space for all our discomforts to coexist. It may open the possibility that everyone's perspective has a place in the story, and when that happens, maybe we won't have to shout so loudly to be heard. Living with (and *as*) contradiction is the nature of Yoga. It is all in each of us, and a resilient approach doesn't exile any of those parts. Instead, it cultivates the capacity for togetherness within. When we can hold more of ourselves within, we find a greater willingness to hold all things together and at once outside of ourselves. We find greater capacity, more space, more consent, more acceptance—or we may not, and we can have space to hold that too.

The Complexity of Autonomy and Sovereignty

In these times of fierce individuation and "bootstrap" culture, we tout the myth that anything is possible if we just work hard enough. It's easy to confuse the achievements and successes that map the points of our story with growth and learning that refine our character and lay the path of resilience. Maturity is measured by this distinction: the evolution from attainment to acquiescence. From a mature vantage point, we lean into the offerings of each experience without a set of demands that require the outer world to meet us in any particular way. We step into the experience of autonomy (defined as "personal independence") and move through the world in sovereignty (complete independence and self-rule). We continue to be shaped and sculpted by our experiences, but rather than be a passive recipient, we step into an active allowing and awareness. I would argue that this is the most accurate definition of enlightenment: the freedom (lightening) of the load of our separation and the full acknowledgment of our absolute self-responsibility.

This state of being leaves room for error and faltering. It opens us fully to the lived experience of each moment and invites us to respond from the knowing that arises from inside. It does not disengage us from our lives, but it does (as the Yogic texts repeat often) allow us to move from a place of detachment/nonattachment. Our experiences are no longer in service to our identity, but rather the cultivation and refinement of our identity shifts into service of every experience. We begin to honor the roles that we have been entrusted with in our respective lives, and we show up fully, always curious as to where and how more fullness can be accessed. We are no longer chasing the "perfect" lives of others but surrender to the blundering and meandering lives we have been offered.

This is not to say that in maturity we do not seek or act to make change, to defend, or to fight. On the contrary, the mature approach responds to injustice from a place that isn't attached to winning or losing but is in alignment with the cause, the idea, or the change itself. Resilience teaches us that things don't always work out like we would choose, but they still always work out if we let them. Maturity is the experience of letting things work out. It recognizes that *everything* is out of our control and leans into the experience as it is offered without the cushion of security or requirement. The only outcome maturity desires is to be shaped by the experience rather than to be the shaper of it. Maturity allows for the results of our choices that are not immediately known and enables our contributions to extend well beyond a moment in time or our personal desires.

Maturity and resilience are long-term games, as they involve time that extends before us and beyond us and isn't dependent upon us. In the long-term view, we recognize the importance of actions that ripple out and ahead of us. We see that our choices impact more than the immediate surroundings and relations and, if offered wisely, may have impact well beyond anything that we know. This length of time invites us to willingly slow down our response time to a planetary rhythm rather than the exhausting breakneck speed of modern life. Slowing down allows space and attention. It allows listening to something bigger than our small story, and it unravels us from our ideas of self-importance. Slowing down removes us from the role of hero or villain and offers instead the opportunity to be shaped by what compels us. Slowing down puts us in touch with the long term and reminds us of our place in it. When we act from this awareness, every act is a service, and every act is more. This is the essence of living Yoga. The pulse of resilience. The power that we hold.

Practice and Application

Feel and Observe: Take a slow walk. Rather than walk on or over the ground, walk with it. Become aware of the ground beneath your feet as you take each step. Feel the experience of connecting, heel to toe, with the surface on which you are walking. Observe the relationship between your body and the ground beneath you.

Inquiry: How does your perception of the world change when you slow down? How are you in a relationship with your life right now?

Movement: Sit or lie down on the floor. Become aware of every part of your body that touches the surface beneath you. From within, soften and open to this connection. As if you are liquid, filling the container that the ground provides, allow yourself to puddle into the support. Notice this movement, imperceptible to the external eye yet present and unfolding from within.

Āsana and Energetics Suggestions:

Explore these āsanas as a resource for greater presence, renewal, and restoration (prāṇa).

CRP
Legs Up the Wall
Shavāsana

15

Tools and Supports

More and more research is pointing to the importance of the body in resolving our mental, emotional, and intellectual challenges. We can't simply think our way to healing; it must be embodied. Embodiment is essentially the experience of being in the body rather than in our heads, dragging our bodies along for the ride. True embodiment expands our intelligence, it increases our capacity to sustain and heal, and it creates a connection to our innermost truth. Lucky for us, Yoga is a system that has embodiment built into the design. The practice of āsana (seat, to sit with/in) is an invitation to feel and discover, integrate and heal.

This chapter will serve as a guide for observing and discovering how to integrate the theories presented throughout this book into embodied practice. By using the tools of energetics, movement, breath, and meditation, we will have the opportunity to move these ideas from the conceptual and intellectual into the realm of direct experience.

Our bodies are a storehouse of our memories and experiences, and whether or not we realize it, the world has left its mark. Perhaps it is an ache in our hip or a skip in our breath or maybe it's the way we direct our gaze when we feel overwhelmed; whatever it is, our lived experiences are held in our physiology until we bring awareness to it and ultimately choose to integrate it into the whole. According to Yogic theory, the entirety of our being is a complex series of constellated energies that move, effect, initiate, govern, and impact the whole. When these assembled energies are in resonance (or harmony) with each other, we feel *sattwa* (tranquility). When there is agitation, aggravation, or stagnancy within a set of energies or between sets, there is dissonance. These energies in Yoga are referred to as "prāna," as discussed in Chapter 8, and they are omnipresent, essential, and highly impactful. Yoga's sister science, *Āyurveda*, organizes our manifestations of prāna in five categories based on location, function, movement, and governance. These five categories are known collectively as the *prāna vāyus*, which were explored in Chapter 8, and are a subset of *Vāta Doṣha*.

15. Tools and Supports

Let's take a quick look at these concepts in some practical ways, and then learn how we can directly apply them to support our resilience.

Scientifically, "energy" is defined as (1) "the strength and vitality required for sustained physical or mental activity"; (2) "the power derived from the utilization of physical or ... [mental activity], especially to provide light or heat to work machines"; and (3) that which is required "to perform work" (Lexico, "Energy," n.p.). Energy is expressed in a multitude of measurable ways, such as heat, light, and activity, as well as many immeasurable ways, like emotion, thought, inspiration, and connection. It exists in manifest form as kinetic energy, or energy in motion, as well as in unmanifest form, known as "potential energy," which is energy possessed by virtue of its position relative to others, stressors within itself, electrical charge, etc., but not yet made manifest.

The Yogic approach to energy holds the same basic principles as Western science but changes the lens through which it is viewed. The practices of Yoga are designed to develop awareness and sensitivity to the various expressions of energy within our bodies and to offer conscious and engaged choice as a means to utilize them. In Yoga, āsana and prāṇāyāma are two of the main and most familiar ways that we harness, shape, direct, and move energy.

Using Yoga in this way requires that we become sensitive to how energy feels and moves in our bodies. This book offers practices that will enable us to dive deeply into the discovery of energy alongside the work of using our minds to understand and explore that information.

"Energy" is an often used buzzword in modern Yoga classes, but to what extent do we really know what it means, how it feels, what it affects, and how we can use it?

The main ways that Yoga defines "energy" (and the ways we will be working with here) are:

1. *Shakti*—the feminine force of action and manifestation; the vibration of the source that underlies all thought, action, and inspiration. Often translated as "power" or "impulse."
2. Prāṇa—first unit. The initial spark that generated physical form, thought, action, and expression. The animating force that expresses *shakti*. Often associated with the breath but also includes all animate and inanimate expressions of energy.

Energy is simply this: the expression of or potential for action. In short, *everything* is energy. The densest physical formations are slowly vibrating forms of energy (seemingly inert but still measurable in action), and the most etheric spaces, such as the air or another gaseous substance, have the most quickly vibrating molecules of energy.

How Your Choices Impact Your Energy

Your system is a never-ending network of energetic potential, action, and interaction. The energy within your system encompasses the entire spectrum, ranging from the slowly vibrating energies (those that create density, stability, depression, form, groundedness, and lethargy) all the way to the quickly vibrating energies (those that are the source of creativity, inspiration, imagination, and oftentimes groundlessness, anxiety, overwhelmingness, and confusion, thought, and emotion). This spectrum of energy is not something we can see or touch. Energy is something we feel. Rather than see it, we measure its results. Energy affects us and impacts the way we move through the world and the ways in which we experience life.

To approach your Yoga practice energetically, you are agreeing to engage with what *is* rather than what you think should be. An energetic approach to practice requires us to relinquish the need to control the experience and outcomes and instead surrender to the process of feeling whatever shows up. When we surrender the need to control our practice, we open the door to refining our sensitivity, addressing what we discover skillfully, and experiencing Yoga and resilience directly. This approach transfers powerfully into our lives as the courage to surrender control and show up to what is from a place of embodiment and intention.

The first and most essential step in the process of energetic practice is the tool of self-awareness. When we are self-aware, we have access to autonomy and sovereignty, and we take responsibility for knowing where we are and what we need. From a place of self-awareness and embodiment, we are actively feeling into our bodies, feeling beneath our thoughts and worries, and gaining access to more and more subtle messages of our experiences. We begin to recognize the signs of imbalance before that imbalance becomes a full-blown crisis, and in doing so, we avoid the steeper climb needed to return to ease and harmony. Getting to know ourselves and being aware of our own needs is a process that gets easier with practice, though it will always be a perpetual challenge influenced by our environment, culture, relationships, and personal identity. When we learn that the most essential part of practice begins and ends with thorough self-observation, we become more attuned to these nuances in our day-to-day lives. We are always in an energetic experience, even when we are typing madly on a keyboard, stuck behind a screen. Energy is omnipresent. It is also subtle. It's not always evident unless we look. It takes slowing down and becoming more sensitive to truly get to know it. To live a life in Yoga, we recognize that our lives are bigger than only our individual expressions. We begin to see that our choices ripple, and that whether we know it or not, our choices are a service that we are offering to others, to our communities, and even our planet. It is imperative that we become aware and sensitive to our own energy in order to effectively support the energy around us. When we recognize that we are making an impact and contributing to the meaning of everything, we are called into radical self-responsibility. We recognize that we are not as confined or defined as we perceive ourselves to be. In our Yoga practice, that means that we become less and less dependent upon outside eyes, adjustments, or diagnoses. We learn how to feel the subtle expressions of our postures as the easeful or challenging expressions of energy, and we can choose to explore our sensations more deeply or change directions. When we begin practicing in this way, we may never approach our mat the same way again.

Energetics in Āsana

Every time we practice Yoga, we are affecting our energy. Because energy is all things, everything we do has an effect. *Āsanas* are especially accessible and potent ways to shape, change, and move energy because that is their purpose. The construction of a form with our bodies is only part of the equation affecting our energy. Intention and awareness also play a huge role. When energy is altered without intent or awareness, the spectrum of impact is broad and unpredictable. However, when we learn, even just a little, about the function, location, and movement of energy inside our systems, we are able to make choices about the how, why, and what we practice and, in turn, direct our practices toward the most beneficial outcomes.

Prāṇa

Let's talk about prāṇa for a moment. As mentioned earlier in this chapter and in preceding chapters, prāṇa is life-force energy. I like to describe our relationship with prāṇa and the ways we can access it with the metaphor of a racehorse and a jockey. The racehorse represents any action or potential action, such as taking a breath or eating a piece of kale, and the jockey represents the life-force energy that rides upon the action. So, prāṇa, in essence, rides upon the breath or a piece of kale. It is the life-giving energy of existence in manifest form, and it is coupled with the building blocks of energy as they exist in our world. With practice, we can recognize the subtle difference between prāṇa and the more gross forms of energy, like the breath or our food, and we can work with the ways that we shape and move prāṇa to provide the outcomes we desire. Every posture we take, every move we make is a container through which we are moving and shaping energy.

When we practice āsana with wisdom and awareness, we can choose forms to help us open up, stabilize, inspire, or release. We learn how to skillfully move and shape our energy within our postures rather than relying on our physical efforts alone to make an impact. The methods that I suggest utilize your āsana practice as a way to invite more awareness and harmony not only into your physical practice but also into your life off the mat.

The prerequisite requirement for this kind of practice is a basic ability to observe and cultivate a felt sense of where you are energetically in the moment. Once you have an understanding of that, you will be able to accurately determine what practices are needed to bring insight, support, and ease to your time both on and off the mat. This approach also requires slowing down the practice significantly. My suggestions will eliminate much of the extraneous movement within and between *āsanas* and instead encourage you to feel more in less postures. The physical practice (coupled with our breath) will be a tool to guide your energy toward its fullest capacity, and from this place, we can ease into expanding that capacity beyond its current limits. The majority of the suggestions in the Practice and Application sections focus on spending time on the simple act of self-observation. This act is essential to empowering your understanding and experience of your practice energetically. Please do not skip it.

Steps to an Energetically
Focused Āsana Practice.

1. Determine your current energetic state (self-observation).
2. Determine what is needed to bring harmony to your system (*sattwa*).
3. Choose an energetic focus for your practice (āsana and prāṇāyāma).

4. Practice slowly with ease, steadiness, and awareness.
5. *Always* end with *Śhavāsana*.

Prāṇa Vāyus

Here we will expand on the topic that we began exploring in Chapter 8. In *Āyurveda*, the sister science to Yoga, there are three main categories of biological energy, called *"Doṣha"* in Sanskrit. As referred to in Chapter 8, these are called *"Vāta," "Pitta,"* and *"Kapha."* In more intermediate-level understanding, each of these three categories are further divided into five subcategories. For the purposes of exploring prāṇa, we will be looking only at the five subcategories of *Vāta Doṣha* known as the *"prāṇa vāyus."* If you desire to develop a deeper understanding of the remaining two *doṣhas* and their subsets, please see the appendix for additional resources.

The *prāṇa vāyus* provide a deeper and more thorough understanding of prāna and how it operates within us physically, mentally, emotionally, and spiritually. The word *"vāyu"* means "wind," and the *prāṇa vāyus*, like the wind, help us to understand the way energy moves and functions within the whole of our system, much like an internal energetic weather, and also the ways that *vāyus* cooperate with the energies of our world. As mentioned above, the *vāyus* are characterized uniquely by location, movement, and the force that they govern. It is important to understand that these subdivisions are not linear but rather are all constantly overlapping and interacting. Much like our physical systems in which the heart and lungs are interdependent in their function such that the health of one (or lack thereof) directly impacts the health of the other, the *vāyus* are perpetually in concert with each other. The function of one *vāyu* will have an impact on all the other four, and just as each of us are one of a kind, the function and expression of our individual *vāyus* are also unique.

We will discuss each of the *vāyus* in detail, along with examples of *āsanas* and pranayamas that help to enliven or subdue or balance their forces. The five *prāṇa vāyus* are as follows: *apāna vāyu, prāṇa vāyu, samāna vāyu, udāna vāyu,* and *vyāna vāyu.* Please reference and apply these understandings outlined below when designing your practices and applications for each of the preceding chapters, and remember, you are an everchanging entity, never the same in any given moment. Therefore, you will need to bring the process of self-observation to each practice and utilize these descriptions and suggestions to create a unique experience that meets your needs every time you practice.

Apāna Vāyu

Apāna vāyu is the energy that is located and moves from the pelvis to the root. It governs organs of elimination. It is an eliminative force. This energy moves downward and outward.

The postures and breathing techniques relative to *apāna vāyu* are focused on the grounding and eliminative force of energy. The awareness is centered in the low abdomen and pelvis, down the legs to the feet. The action moves waste energy and toxicity down and out of the system so that it can be released, resulting in the purification of body, mind, and psychospiritual functioning.

THE ENERGY OF GROUNDING AND LETTING GO. When energy moves down and out through *apāna vāyu*, it allows us to release physical waste as well as patterns that no longer serve us. It influences physical, mental, emotional, and spiritual release and the energies associated with elimination, which can manifest as the willingness and action of letting go of those things that no longer serve us.

Practices that release stagnant energy are also practices that ground and root you in the world. When your energetic system is holding on to contamination, waste, or residue, it robs you of your ability to be fully present and vital in the moment. Weak *apāna vāyu* will have you cycling back to past experiences, mired in worry and anxiety, feeling stuck and stagnant, and even depressed. Activating and empowering the energy of letting go helps eliminate unwanted waste from the body as well as outmoded feelings, ideas, and thoughts. Strong *apāna vāyu* mobilizes past experiences and helps to clear remnants of the old thoughts, memories, and impressions that are no longer serving the health of the system. You can utilize these grounding practices when you are feeling overwhelmed or if you find yourself repeating unsupportive patterns over and over. *Apāna vāyu* also supports the cleansing and release of the physical systems of elimination (colon, bladder, reproductive organs, etc.).

ĀSANAS[1] TO SUPPORT *APĀNA VĀYU*: The Energy of Grounding and Releasing. Standing postures that direct energy down your torso toward your feet and into the ground include:

Tadāsana
Utkatāsana

---

1. I will be using the Sanskrit names of the *āsanas* to reduce confusion. Graphics accompany posture names to clarify the descriptions.

Uttānāsana
Vīrabhadrāsana II
Prasārita Pādottānāsana
Mālāsana

Forward folds with emphasis on energy dropping into the pelvis and releasing down the legs to the ground include:

Upaviṣhṭa Koṇasana
Paschimottānāsana
Baddha Koṇāsana
Adho Mukha Śhvānāsana
Bālāsana

Lengthen exhalations both on your mat and off. Smooth and refine the breath while working to make the exhale as much as twice as long as your inhale.

Samāna Vāyu

Samāna vāyu is the energy in the abdomen centered around the naval. It governs organs of digestion. It is the force of assimilation, digestion, and balancing. Movement is from the periphery to the center.

In our modern world, we typically don't live in our bodies. The majority of our living is done from our brain. Our bodies have become either something that we drag around behind us or float above. We all know that our brain doesn't have all the answers and most often is the main cause of our suffering and confusion, yet we continually allow this small fraction of our self to control the whole.

Practices designed to gather the energy that has been hijacked by our thoughts and the environment and bring it into our center where we can digest it fully work to strengthen *samāna vāyu*, the force of digestion and assimilation. By sending wastes to be eliminated down to *apāna* and retaining energies that can support our growth and inspiration, *samāna* helps us to assimilate all that we take in (from food to media to beliefs) so that we don't continue to repeat our undigested experiences. Strong energy in this place helps us to manage the whole of our lives more skillfully because once we have digested our experiences, we learn the lessons we are meant to learn, and we are able to bring those lessons with us into the future and let go of the necessity to repeat them.

Working with the energy in this area also supports taking in nutrients and information and being nourished by it. If we are not able to take in and fully digest our experiences and assimilate the lessons that each of these experiences offer, we struggle. When we are able to digest our lives, our thoughts become clearer, our bodies healthier, and though we are still faced with many challenges, we feel more able to meet them. We work with the energy in this area when we feel scattered or overwhelmed and unable to find a steady center.

ĀSANAS TO SUPPORT SAMĀNA VĀYU: The Energy of Assimilation and Digestion. Postures that gather attention and energy into the abdomen include:

> *Utkatāsana*
> *Nāvāsana*
> *Śhalabhāsana*
> *Adho Mukha Śhvānāsana*
> *Bālāsana*

Twisting Postures that are concentrated in the abdomen include:

> *Parivṛtta Pārśhvakoṇāsana*
> *Ardha Matsyendrāsana*
> *Jaṭhara Parivartanāsana*

Focus your breath in the belly. Use diaphragmatic breathing and also a balanced breath cycle, called *"sama vritti"* in Sanskrit.

Prāṇa Vāyu

Prāṇa vāyu is energy located in the chest. Its movement is inward and upward. It governs the heart and lungs. It is the force of inspiration, vitalization, and renewal.

The energy of *prāṇa vāyu* propels us toward growth on all levels. On a physical level, this is the energy of cellular renewal; on a mental level, this is the energy of intelligence; and, on a spiritual level, this is the energy of evolution. This energy inspires us to grow into the very essence of who we are meant to be and elevates us out of mundane life and assists us in seeing our full potential.

With lives inundated by stimuli, activity, and responsibility, it is common for this energy to be deficient, resulting in the feeling of being drained or exhausted. When you are stressed, overwhelmed, and busy, energy in this area becomes depleted.

15. Tools and Supports

When *prāṇa vāyu* is full, you feel a sense of vitality and inspiration and maintain your focus easily. You feel fully engaged in the unfolding of your life, alive and present in your experiences without distraction or confusion. Working with *prāṇa vāyu* enables you to find deep, nourishing stillness within as a source of vitality and vigor. Movements to support *prāṇa vāyu* focus on drawing energy into your heart center and expanding the space and the breath in this area. Energy that is gathered in this area will help sustain and inspire you. This energy activates the intelligence of your heart (different from mental intelligence), which is sourced from felt-sense experience rather than logic and analysis and is perfect for seeking guidance and creative and generative solutions.

Increased energy in this area will support meditative practice as well because you will be nourished by quiet and stillness rather than distracted or uncomfortable. Strong *prāṇa vāyu* results in your mind and body becoming calmer and more comfortable. The movement of energy will expand through the chest and the space of the heart, and you will get a true feeling of what it means to have a heart-centered practice.

ĀSANAS TO SUPPORT *PRĀṆA VĀYU*: The Energy of Revitalization and Renewal. These include postures that gather energy in the center of the chest.

Lateral and side-body-opening postures that support breath moving through the chest include:

Vīrabhadrāsana II
Trikonāsana
Adho Mukha Śhvānāsana

Gentle backbending postures that direct energy into the chest and upward to the crown include:

Setu Bandha Sarvāṅgāsana
Śhalabhāsana
Sphinx

Restorative postures that support renewal include:

Legs Up the Wall
CRP

Breath that is focused on expanding and opening the space of the chest, i.e., long inhalations, pausing at the top of inhalation, and expanding prāṇa fully in the chest.

Udāna Vāyu

Udāna vāyu is located in the throat. Its movement is up and out. It governs the throat and all of the structures and glands within it. It is the force of expression and enthusiasm.

Focusing on *udāna vāyu* opens the space of the throat, neck, and upper chest. The effect of full energy in this area is that you will feel more expressive, more excited to share, and more excited to create.

We are all artists of our own lives, and the energy that supports us in our creations is governed by this area of movement. Our desire to express our joy and creativity on all levels is centralized here. When we feel dull, uninspired, or muted in our expression, we work to build the energy of *udāna vāyu*. The location and movement of this energy support our creative force and enthusiasm for life. When we activate energy where *udāna vāyu* is located, we find our individual voice in the world, and we are excited to share it. We are able to speak our truth with sensitivity and compassion, and we move in the direction of what inspires us.

Weak *udāna vāyu* results in repression and a lack of self-expression. This energy can become weak after periods of "holding your tongue" or silencing your thoughts/opinions/feelings. It also weakens when our desires to create are stifled. Life situations in which sharing clearly and honestly is prevented affects this energy. Building the energy of *udāna vāyu* raises your joie de vivre.

ĀSANAS TO SUPPORT UDĀNA VĀYU: The Energy of Expression and Enthusiasm. Postures that open the space of the throat include:

Chakravākāsana
Trikonāsana
Adho Mukha Śhvānāsana
Setu Bandha Sarvāṅgāsana
Matsyāsana

Vyāna Vāyu

Vyāna vāyu is located everywhere. It governs circulation and distribution. Its movement is from center to periphery. It is the force of circulation and integration.

The movement of *vyāna vāyu* is circulatory. Very much like the cardiovascular system of our physical bodies, this energy movement is designed to distribute the vital energy of prāṇa throughout our entire system. When energy is refined within the container of the body, it is *vyāna vāyu* that takes that energy throughout our system to where it is needed. Therefore, we say it is located everywhere, within and outside the body. The force of circulation allows stuck and stagnant energy to flow. It circulates nourishment throughout the entire body as well as supports the distribution of energy from one space to another. In doing so, the building and refining of this energy enlivens you and enables you to step into the flow of life. When things are flowing smoothly, you are able to expand yourself to the fullest capacity that you are capable of achieving.

Work with *vyāna vāyu* if you are feeling stuck or unable to go with the flow in your life. When you feel resistant to movement or change, moving energy in this way will help free you from your constrictions and open up the flow of greater possibility. This energy assists all the other energies in the system to function and distribute optimally. The emphasis of this *vāyu* is on building fluidity and capacity. Because this practice will enliven and invigorate you, it's best that it is not used as a winding-down practice or done in the evening.

In the moments of life when we feel stuck and our energy is low, there is a resistance to moving through our experiences. We can easily get caught in a pattern of behavior that causes us to feel like we are out of the flow of life. Practicing *vyāna vāyu* assists the physical body in increasing its capacity, stretching the sense of energy to the edges of our perception. When we increase the felt sense of our periphery, we are able to increase our capacity to sustain, grow, and engage. A focus on *vyāna vāyu* helps you to return to the flow that is bigger than you perceive yourself to be. It supports the integration of lessons and experiences and ownership over the whole of our lives. This results in enjoyment of the events and experiences we encounter and the ability to generate lessons from our losses.

Āsanas to Support Vyāna Vāyu: The Energy of Circulation and Integration. Postures that extend your central energy outward to the periphery include:

> *Chakravākāsana*
> *Vīrabhadrāsana* II
> *Adho Mukha Śhvānāsana*
> CRP
> *Tadāsana*
> *Śhavāsana*

149

Use an expansive, full breath that brings breath into the periphery of the body. Complete breathing.

Practice with Prana

When we fully understand the impact and possibility that we can access by applying energetic principles to our āsana practice, our relationship to our practice changes. In order to reap the rewards of our intellectual understanding, we must run them in and through our physical bodies. Using the principles of the *prāṇa vāyus*, we can experiment with cultivating a deeper connection to our bodies and, therefore, more fully integrate the concepts and experiences of resilience. All these principles are merely theoretical until you begin to experience the effects for yourself. Whether you are a Yoga teacher or a curious student, energy is meant to be experienced and not simply studied.

When you begin to have direct experience of energetics in your āsana practice, you can align your internal experiences with the knowledge and intellectual understanding offered in the preceding chapters. Over time, these explorations will expand beyond your Yoga mat and cushion and truly become your own. The result may be that you discover unique and even more powerful ways to have an energetic impact on your body and in your life.

Please remember that what we do on our mat is simply a reflection of our life in the world, and conversely, the ways we move and the feelings that surface through our Yoga practice are a direct reflection of the lives we are living (and have lived). If we are stuck or uncomfortable in our Yoga, we can observe those same discomforts and stagnations in our lives. Bringing our Yoga and our resilience into full awareness requires direct experience and will ultimately help us to make big shifts in our lives, our relationships, our communities, and even our planet.

I hope that this overview provides a road map to follow in your own explorations and that you will take them into your body and mind until they become real for you. It is from this place of direct experience that insights and discoveries will emerge, and when put into direct action in your life, this knowledge can greatly benefit you and those around you.

Final tip: *keep a journal*! Become an attentive observer of your own experience and record your discoveries and disappointments. No one knows you better than yourself. Keep track of your experiences in āsana and in life and watch how the practice unfolds.

16

Conclusion

Caminante, no hay camino,
se hace camino al andar.
Al andar se hace el camino ....

Pathmaker, there is no path,
You make the path by walking.
By walking you make the path ...
["Life Isn't a Straight Line," n.p.].
—Antonio Machado, translation
by David Whyte

The Yoga of resilience is a practice and an experience of living life fully. It is not a shortcut to balance or ease, nor does it promise happy end ings. The Yoga of resilience is a path of refinement, polishing, reflection, review, and return, over and over again. It will meet us wherever we are and ask us to remember what we are capable of. It will direct us to the tools that we have available at any given moment and help us remember how to use them. Most likely, this path will not change your life, though every thing in your life may change.

The Yoga of resilience is an approach to living exactly where you are while keeping a toe in where you've been and with your finger pointing in the direction of where you are going. It is an opportunity to weave all the parts of yourself together into a holy, imperfect whole. It can open our eyes and our hearts and make space for potential to emerge without the requirement that our circumstances change. It is a path of accountability and responsibility, not a burden but an opportunity to expand our capac ity and show up for "more" in our families, our relationships, our commu nities, and our world.

This path is not one of salvation or even respite. It will not make the hard things easier, and it will not make the difficult things disappear. The path of the Yoga of resilience is a reality check, planting you squarely where you are, and offering up the inquiry, "Now, what am I going to do with this?" The practice is one of learning and failing, of celebration and sorrow, and of awareness and integrity. Most likely, if you choose it, you already know what's required of you, and you are willing to move bravely into the mysterious unknown with openness to the potential that you cannot see. It is the path of courage in its original meaning: from the heart. It names what it sees, accesses vulnerability as strength, and holds arms open to include all perspectives.

This path is one of internal resonance rather than external expectation. It tunes our ears to hear the quiet but unrelenting bass notes of what's "more," and it identifies the places where there is dissonance as well as the space into which we can share our song. The Yoga of resilience builds capacity for what is and what is to come, without requiring any measurable understanding of what that is. It calls forth the full spectrum of experience to be included and celebrates each and every moment in which we surrender into the fullness of being alive. The practice and experience expand our ability to hold more, while holding no category or judgment. When we live the Yoga of resilience, we conspire to be a part of the whole, consciously and with agency, prodding our sleeping awareness awake, challenging us to show up unless we don't, and then inviting us again, and again, and again.

Yoga and resilience are not something you can learn. It's who you are. You can't fail at being yourself, you can't fail at Yoga, and you can't fail at resilience. You will arrive exactly as you are meant to, and you will emerge as more of whatever you discover along the way. This path will not perfect you, and it will not heal you, but it will allow you to engage with what you discover. The parts that are uniquely you will be welcomed in and encouraged to share in the extraordinary expression of your individuation. You will be the treasure and the offering. You will be the parts and the whole.

The Yoga of resilience offers no answers, only more questions in an ever-deepening journey of inquiry and review. There will be no bad discoveries on this path, only a growing collection of insights and recognitions that lead you home to yourself over and over again. To be resilient is an invitation to be fully present, engaged, and accountable for what we bring in our process of becoming. It makes the path by walking, and there are no shortcuts. It brings us over and over again to the intersection of choice, calling us to bring forth our lessons and foibles, our forgetting and remembering. As in life, resilience requires us to choose a direction but does not guarantee that our choice will get us where we desire to go.

Yoga and resilience alike are tools for navigating the journey; without them, we may be stuck but never for long. It calibrates our compass inward, orienting us to a knowing that has never been far away but has been hard to find. Yoga and resilience are a return to trust, to power, to authenticity, and though the path may meander through thickets of challenge and pain, it always leads us home in the end. I hope that this contemplation and amalgamation have been of use. I hope that the suggestions and the tools you have found here will serve you wherever you are in this life. It is by no means complete. You are discovering your path, and I pray that this book has been another tool to add to your arsenal of support.

It has been a weighty honor and a raucous celebration to bear witness to so many journeys in my almost 30 years as a student and teacher of this path. I have overwhelming gratitude toward every student who took a chance, every aspiring teacher who gave my opinions a second thought, every one with whom I butted heads and those who butted back. The best I can offer you is my integrity and my unwavering commitment to continue to walk this path beside you. I will be here. I'm not going anywhere.

Thanks and Acknowledgments

Despite all the words, there are never enough in the end. I am deeply grateful for every teacher that has crossed my path. Mrs. Smith and Mrs. Misener, you taught me that words have power and meaning and that to say them wasn't enough: you have to live into them to be heard.

Rod Stryker, Douglas Brooks, and the many white male teachers of the Western Tantric lineage: you have taught me to lean into the sharp edges of growth, and guided me to discover that the "truth" of this practice is neither masculine nor authoritarian. It was always too much and never enough, it was always brilliant and artful, and there was always more, even if you didn't know it yourself.

Angela Farmer, you showed me that the goddess has power and she lives in my body. You showed me the fierce tenderness of a woman who has been rocked on the waves of this world and still swims naked in the sea. Your embodied wisdom is unparalleled, and your willingness to articulate it is a gift.

To all my heart friends, especially Serena Crawford, you know who you are. I would not be here without your believing mirrors, reminding me of the capacity that I often forget.

To Kelsey Burke and the Vira Bhava Yoga crew (students, teachers, mentors, friends), this would not have been possible without *you*. So, here is the book you've been asking for all these years. I hope it was worth the wait.

To Amy Smith, teacher, poet, partner in crime. What an honor. You have an amazing gift of redirection that inspires confidence when I feel stuck and that pushes me to be more. You have a patience as wide as the ocean and an unwavering nature that anchors on stormy seas. Thank you for the reads, the edits, the feedback, the encouragement. If this book speaks, it's because you were willing to be engaged in the conversation for the entire journey. I bow in the deepest gratitude and respect.

Thanks and Acknowledgments

To my children, Dharma and Pippa. The biggest blessing of this incarnation was that two amazing daughters traversed time and space to find me. Thank you for loving me at my worst, celebrating me at my best. Thank you for being my heart, my soul, and my constant inspiration. I am overjoyed to watch you both become the powerful, intelligent, beautiful, and resilient women that you are. What a gift.

To my parents. All my life, you said "yes" to my wild and crazy dreams. You said "yes" to poetry when everyone else's kids were becoming teachers and lawyers. You said "yes" to my hard lessons and my long journeys away from myself. And you always, always opened your hearts to let me come home. I have never been without a team of unquestioning love and support. Mom, my hero. Dad, my idol. This book was forged in the fire of the end of days. Thank you for inviting me in and letting me stay for a lifetime.

Index of *Āsanas* with Brief Instruction

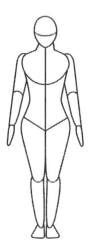

***Tadāsana*:** Stand firmly rooted on the ground with both feet parallel. Feel weight descending into your heels and space rising up through the vertebrae of the spine. Feel yourself extending in both directions simultaneously. Broaden through the chest and feel your shoulders relax into their sockets. Arms at your sides, rotate to turn the palms forward. Land in this shape.

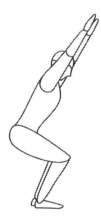

***Utkatāsana*:** Find a strong stance with feet parallel and spine long. Chest open and shoulders relaxed. Slowly and with awareness, press firmly into the feet and begin to drop the pelvis down and back as if moving to sit in a chair. Stop the progression of movement when you are at the limit of your strength, then raise your arms overhead, upper arms parallel to your ears (if possible). Lengthen the spine, feeling your sitting bones release back and down toward the pull of gravity and the tiny hook of your tailbone curve upwards toward your navel, engaging the strength in your low belly and core. Broaden through the chest and relax the shoulders. To come out of

157

this form, press into the feet firmly and straighten the knees to return to standing.

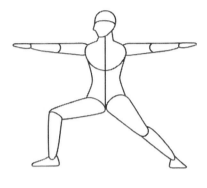

Vīrabhadrāsana II: Stand with feet in a wide stance. Turn your right foot to face your toes forward, and parallel the left foot to the back edge of your mat (toes facing the left side of the room). Press down into both legs and feet, and slowly begin to bend your right knee. Go as far as your strength allows (without bending the knee beyond the ankle). Keep the back leg extended and strong. Feel the torso rise up from the pelvis with the chest facing the left. Lift and out-stretch both arms, reaching the right arm forward in the direction of the right toes and the left arm backward in the direction of the left leg. Work to bring your arms parallel to the floor (palms can be face up or down) and seek a steady strength while neither overworking nor under-working. Rotate the neck to gaze out over the right hand. Land here for a few breaths. To come out of this pose, release the arms. Press the right leg straight and return to a wide-legged standing position. Repeat on the opposite side.

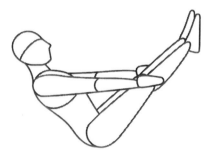

Nāvāsana: From a seated position on the floor, gently lean back toward the back of the pelvis and place both feet on the floor in front of you with knees bent. From the back of the pelvis, lengthen up through the spine, relax the shoulders into the back, and firm the abdomen. Slowly as you are able, lift one foot at a time off the floor until both calves are parallel to the floor beneath you. You can bring your arms behind you and place palms on the floor to support the lift of the legs, or if you feel able, you can extend both arms forward parallel to your lifted lower legs. Maintain stable strength and lower the legs when the shape becomes too challenging.

To release this pose, return the feet to the floor, and release into an easy seated position.

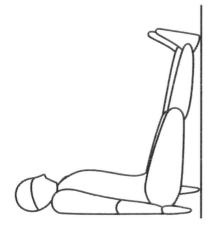

Legs Up the Wall: Sit on the floor as close to a wall as you are able. Turn the torso to either the right or left so that the hips face the direction of the torso and the hip closest to the wall is perpendicular to the wall. Slowly use your hand and arm to lower yourself down to the floor and rotate the hips to reach the legs up the wall. Extend both legs as straight as is comfortable while the torso is lying flat on the floor with spine extended. Rest here, feeling the tops of the femur bones sinking into the hip sockets, with the full length of the spine and the back of the head resting on the floor. To release the pose, pull both knees toward the chest and roll to one side. From here, use your hands to press you gently up to a seated position.

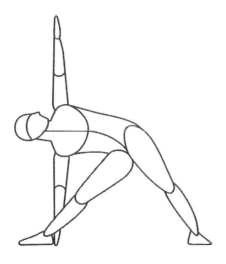

Trikoṇāsana: From standing, come to a wide-leg stance. Turn your right foot to face your toes forward, and parallel the left foot to the back edge of your mat (toes facing the left side of the room). Press down into both feet to generate strength and stability, while keeping both legs straight with knees unlocked. Raise both arms parallel to the floor. Lengthening the side of the body and waist, reach out and over your right leg, extending the right arm as far as you can reach toward the right. At the point of your fullest reach, drop the right arm and hand down and place the hand on the thigh, shin, ankle, or top of the foot (or onto a block if available). Reach the left arm straight up to the

159

sky, feeling both arms extending away from the spine in opposite directions, opening the space of the chest. Turn the gaze directly forward. Careful not to overextend either knee, the hips, or shoulders. Take care not to push beyond your current capacity. Stay anchored to your back foot. When you are ready to come out of the pose, gently bend your front knee and use the strength in your legs and core to raise yourself back to center. Repeat on the other side.

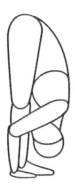

Uttānāsana: Stand firmly rooted on the ground with both feet parallel. Lengthening the spine and, leading with the heart, fold forward from the hips and reach your arms toward your toes (it's okay if they don't touch). If the legs or back are uncomfortable, bend the knees until you find an accessible shape with the heart below the hips. Allow the arms to release toward the floor and rest your hands wherever feels comfortable. Remain here for a few breaths. To come out of this form, bend the knees and engage the strength of your abdomen and core, rise up with a long spine, and return to standing.

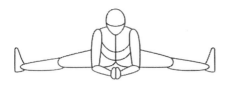

Upaviṣṭa Koṇasana: From a seated position on the floor (or in your bed), extend both legs out to the sides. If the backs of the legs are tight and/or if the lower back is feeling discomfort, you can lift the hips and pelvic floor up onto a support (pillow, blanket, block, bolster) and slightly bend the knees. From this position, lift and lengthen the spine and relax the shoulders into the back of the body. Begin to fold forward at the hips, bringing both hands to the floor and walking them gently forward while being mindful of the sensations in your hips, legs, and back. Stop walking the hands forward when you are feeling stretch but not discomfort. Linger here for a few breaths. To come out of the pose, tone the abdomen and lengthen the spine, gently walking your hands back toward your body to get back into a comfortable seated position.

Paschimottānāsana: From a comfortable seated position on the floor (or bed), extend both legs straight out in front of you. If the backs of the

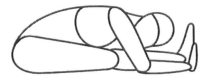

legs are tight and/or if the lower back is feeling discomfort, you can lift the hips and pelvic floor up onto a support (pillow, blanket, block, bolster) and place a slight bend in the knees. From this position, lift and lengthen the spine, relax the shoulders into the back of the body. Leading with the chest and heart with shoulders remaining on the back of the body, begin to fold forward from the hips, slightly tipping the pelvis forward and rolling to the front of the sitting bones. Reach your arms and hands out to rest wherever they land (thighs, shins, feet). Recommit to the length of the spine and feel the abdomen tone but not harden. Soften into the fold and take a few breaths. To come out of the position, tone the abdomen and lengthen the spine, gently walking your hands back toward your body to lift back into a comfortable seated position.

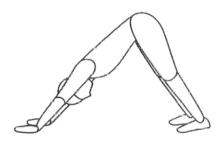

Adho Mukha Śhvānāsana: From all fours (best done on the floor), walk your hands slightly in front of your shoulders and parallel to each other. Press firmly into the full palm and out through the fingers. Curl the toes under and press the hips up into the air, lengthening the spine and bringing the chest to land between the upper arms. Relax the neck and head and release down toward the floor. Hips are lifted. Turn the sitting bones up and slightly back on the diagonal and straighten the legs as much as you are able. Feel the front of the body lengthen with the abdomen toned and the chest broad and the back of the body lengthened and extended. If the lower back or backs of the legs are tight, causing the lower back to round, bend the knees to create more extension. Drop the weight of your heels toward the floor (but they don't have to touch). Push forward and out through the hands, toning the arms, turning the inner elbows toward one another. If the shoulders are tight, you can move the hands farther apart from each other. Allow the shoulders to move into the back of the body and away from the ears. Feel that you are creating the shape of an upside down "V" with your body. To come out of the form, return knees to the floor.

Index of *Āsanas* with Brief Instruction

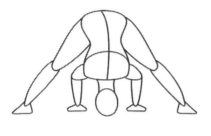

Prasārita Pādottānāsana: Stand with your feet in a wide stance. Stand firmly rooted on the ground with both feet parallel. Lengthening the spine and leading with the heart, fold forward from the hips and reach your arms and hands to the floor (it's okay if they don't touch). If the legs or back are uncomfortable, bend the knees until you find an accessible shape with the heart below the hips. Allow the arms to release toward the floor and rest your hands wherever feels comfortable (on the thighs, shins, ankles, or floor). Remain here for a few breaths. To come out of this form, bend the knees and engage the strength of your abdomen and core, and then rise up with a long spine and return to standing.

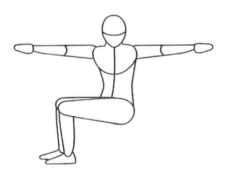

Jaṭhara Parivartanāsana: From a lying position (either on the floor or in your bed), bend the knees and bring them into the abdomen. Keep the shoulders grounded on the surface beneath you, and keeping both knees together, place the right hand on top of the knees and rotate the knees and spine to the right in a gentle twist. Do your best to keep both shoulders anchored and go only as far as is comfortable for your back, knees and hips. Occupy this form for a few breaths, then return to center and repeat on the opposite side. When both sides are completed, rest in CRP.

Ardha Matsyendrāsana: From a seated position, root down through the pelvis and lengthen up through the spine. Extend the left leg forward in front of you, step the right foot over the left leg to the floor. Right knee remains bent and elevated. If comfortable, you can bend the left knee and bring the left foot to the outside of the right hip, but this modification is not necessary to the form. Sitting tall, begin to rotate on the axis of the spine to turn the torso toward the right knee. Place the left hand, forearm or elbow onto the right knee and plant the left hand to the floor behind

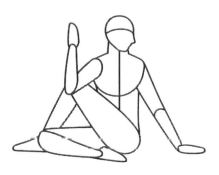

the right hip. Deepen the twist by drawing more of the right side of the abdomen and chest backward and widening the left side of the abdomen and chest toward the lifted right knee. Move into this pose in a way that is most accessible to your body. The head can turn to look over the left shoulder. Be here for a few breaths. To unwind from the pose, turn the gaze forward, gently release the rotation of the torso to return to a neutral position of the spine, then uncross the legs. Take a moment to return to the center before repeating on the opposite side.

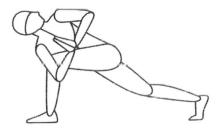

Parivṛtta Pārśhvakoṇāsana: From all fours (or *Adho Mukha Śhvānāsana*), step the right leg forward, placing the right foot between the hands. Lift the torso up into a kneeling position. Extend both arms overhead to lengthen the side of the body and relax both shoulders into the back. Lower the arms and bring the hands together at the center of the chest with palms together. Engage the abdomen and feel stable in the belly. Slowly and with awareness, rotate on the axis of the spine to turn the torso toward the right, possibly resting the left elbow or forearm on top of or to the outside of the right leg. Press into the palms and draw the right shoulder more into the back of the body, feeling the twist engaging at the navel center. If this form feels strong and stable, you can curl your left toes under and extend back through your left leg, lifting your left knee off the ground. A final step, if it feels wise, is to release the right arm in the direction of the floor to the outside of the right leg and extend the right arm forward, parallel to the right ear. To come out of this shape, slowly unwind the rotation of the spine and place both hands back on the floor on either side of the right foot. You can drop the left knee back down to the floor and return to all fours, or you can keep the left knee lifted and step the right leg back into *Adho Mukha Śhvānāsana*.

163

Index of *Āsanas* with Brief Instruction

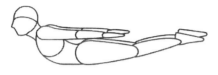

Śhalabhāsana: Lie in a prone position, face down. Feel the belly, chest, and thighs resting on the surface on which you lay. Extend your arms to rest alongside your hips with palms face down. Anchor the tops of the thighs into the floor, and feel your abdomen engage (try drawing your sitting bones back in the direction of your heels and curling the very tip of your tailbone in and up toward your navel center). From here, press into the hands and gently lift the head and chest away from the floor. Keep shoulders on the back of the body and relaxed away from the ears. Keep the chest broad. Gaze to the floor in front of you to keep the back of your neck lengthened. If this position feels sustainable, extend back through the soles of the feet and toes and gently lift your legs up and back away from the floor (not too high). Feel the body anchored to the floor at the navel center and the chest and legs expanding away from the center in opposing directions. After a few breaths here, gently lower the legs, chest, and head back down to the floor and rest.

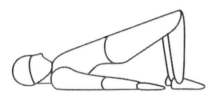

Setu Bandha Sarvāṅgāsana (Bridge): Lie on your back in a supine position with the back of the head, hips, and spine on the floor (or bed). Bend both knees and place the soles of the feet on the floor (or bed). Bring the heels to align with the sitting bones, knees resting over the ankles. Place your hands, palms down, on the floor by your hips. With the shoulders and feet anchored to the floor, press into your hands and lift the spine slowly off the floor beginning at the pelvis, and lifting slowly, only to an accessible point, through the lower back and middle back, keeping your shoulders grounded the whole time. Press gently into the back of the head to maintain length in the cervical spine (neck) and feel the front of the throat remain open as the chest lifts toward the sky. Stay rooted through the soles of both feet. Breathe here for a few cycles of inhalations and exhalations. To release, lower the spine back to the floor beginning at the upper middle back and releasing down to the pelvis. Once the full spine has returned to the floor, you can turn the palms of the hands up to the sky, and step the feet apart into CRP, resting the knees together.

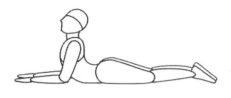

Sphinx: From a prone position with belly and legs on the floor (or bed), gently slide the elbows and forearms to rest on the floor (or bed), lifting the chest and head. Pelvis and legs remain anchored on the floor (or bed), and forearms are parallel to each other. Shoulders rest on the back of the body and the chest broadens. The back of the neck is long, gaze forward. The closer you bring your elbows and forearms to your body, the higher the chest will lift. Respect what your body needs and don't force things. When you are ready to release, widen the elbows to the sides and slowly lower the chest and head back down to the surface on which you are resting.

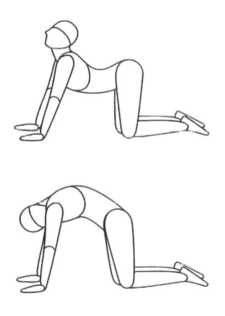

Chakravākāsana (Cat/Cow): From an all-fours position, on an inhale, lengthen the front of the spine by lifting the upper chest forward and gently through the upper arms, lifting the gaze, and drawing the pubic bone back, extending the low belly and slightly tilting the pelvis upward. On an exhale, extend the back of the spine by pressing firmly into the hands and round the spine, drawing the chin to the chest and rounding the spine toward the sky. Drop the sitting bones to the floor and curl the tailbone powerfully in and up. You can move between these two positions for several cycles of the breath. Return to a neutral position of the spine on all fours when you are complete.

Constructive Rest Pose (CRP): Lying prone on your back either on the floor or bed, feel the spine resting on the surface on which you are laying. Also rest the shoulders and the back of the head on the floor (or bed). Bend your knees to approximately over your ankles and place the soles of both feet on the floor. Step the feet out in a position that is wider than

165

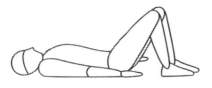

the hips, and allow the knees to fall together, resting against each other. The knees and feet form the shape of a triangle. Rest here. *This pose is a powerful restorative position. It can also be used as a substitute for the Legs up the Wall pose.*

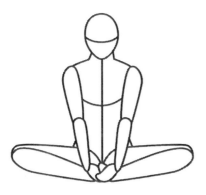

***Baddha Koṇāsana*:** Begin in a comfortable seated position. Bend both knees and touch the soles of the feet together. If this position is uncomfortable on the knees or inner thighs, place a support (blanket, pillow, block, bolster) underneath the knees. If this position is uncomfortable on the lower back, elevate the pelvis onto a support. You can apply both of these modifications together if desired or necessary. From this position, lift and lengthen the spine, relax the shoulders into the back of the body. Leading with the chest and heart with shoulders remaining on the back of the body, begin to fold forward from the hips slightly, tipping the pelvis forward and rolling to the front of the sitting bones. Reach your arms and hands out to rest wherever they land (thighs, shins, feet). Recommit to the length of the spine, and feel the abdomen toned but not hardened. Soften into the fold and take a few breaths. To come out, tone the abdomen and lengthen the spine, gently walking your hands back toward your body to lift back into a comfortable seated position.

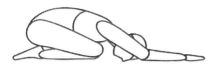

***Bālāsana*:** On the floor or in your bed, sit on your knees (if uncomfortable, place a pillow, block or bolster between your ankles and underneath your pelvis). Fold the torso gently forward over the thighs, with arms outstretched in front of you, and rest. (If you feel discomfort or restriction, you can rest the torso on pillows or a bolster.) Rest here for several breaths. To come up, walk your hands toward your knees and raise your torso off of your thighs.

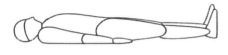

Śhavāsana: Lie flat on your back. Relax completely. Allow arms and hands to rest palms up gently apart from the body. Spread the legs apart and allow the toes to fall outward and heels to turn in. (Feel the whole spine relaxing onto the surface on which you are resting. If the lower back is tense or tight, place a blanket, pillow, or bolster beneath the knees.) Rest here for as long as you can, allowing the breath to soften.

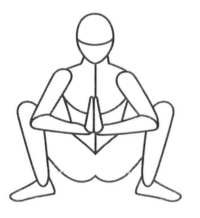

Mālāsana: From a standing position, step your feet out to a point that is slightly wider than hips' width apart and gently and slowly lower yourself down to a squat, resting your pelvis on the support of a block or bolster if needed. Bring the palms together in front of the chest and rest the elbows to the inner knees. (If it is uncomfortable to enter this form from standing, begin on all fours, widen your knees slightly, and walk your hands backward until you are in a squatting position. You can rest the pelvis on a support if needed.) If either position finds the heels lifting uncomfortably off the floor, place a rolled blanket beneath the heels. To come out of this pose, walk hands forward into all fours.

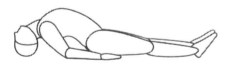

Matsyāsana: *This pose is somewhat challenging to the cervical spine; explore only as far as it feels accessible.* From a supine lying position with the spine resting on the floor (or bed), anchor your shoulders down and bend the elbows to place elbows and forearms on the floor by the waist. Press firmly into elbows and forearms to lift the chest toward the sky and the head off the floor. Gently rest the crown of the head on the floor behind you opening the space of the throat. Careful not to transfer too much weight into the head and instead continue to work the elbows and forearms into the floor to access strength. Be here for a few breaths. *This pose can also be done with support by placing a blanket, pillow, or bolster underneath the upper back (just below the shoulder blades) and resting the back or crown of the head on a blanket.* To come out of this position in either version, turn the gaze upward, and lower the back of the head gently to the floor, releasing the lift of the chest.

Bibliography

Preface

Hoffman, Kent. "With Memorials, Graduations and Other Ceremonies Cancelled Because of COVID, I Went on a Quest for New Rituals." CBC, 8 October 2021. https://www.cbc.ca/radio/docproject/with-memorials-graduations-and-other-ceremonies-cancelled-because-of-covid-i-went-on-a-quest-for-new-rituals-1.6203632. Accessed 4 April 2022.

Introduction

Manchester, Jeanie. "The Epic Ramayana Revealed Through Story & Yoga with Douglas Brooks & Jeanie Manchester." https://www.shambhalamountain.org/program/the-epic-ramayana-revealed-through-story-and-yoga/. Accessed 9 June 2022.

Wilber, Ken. One Taste. Boston & London: Shambhala, 2000.

Chapter 1

Lexico. "Resilient." https://www.lexico.com/en/definition/resilient. Accessed 27 May 2022.

Online Etymology Dictionary. "Stress." https://www.etymonline.com/word/stress. Accessed 4 April 2022.

Satchidananda, Swami. The Yoga Sūtra of Patañjali. Buckingham: Integral Yoga, 2012.

Wikipedia. "Psychological Resilience." Accessed 4 April 2022. https://en.wikipedia.org/wiki/Psychological_resilience.

Chapter 2

National Institute of Mental Health. "I'm So Stressed Out! Fact Sheet." https://www.nimh.nih.gov/health/publications/stress/index.shtml. Accessed 4 April 2022.

Online Etymology Dictionary. "Stress." https://www.etymonline.com/word/stress. Accessed 4 April 2022.

Psychology Today. "Adverse Childhood Experiences." https://www.psychology-today.com/us/basics/adverse-childhood-experiences. Accessed 30 May 2022.

Psychology Today. "Compassion Fatigue." https://www.psychologytoday.com/us/basics/compassion-fatigue. Accessed 30 May 2022.

Psychology Today. "Trauma." https://www.psychologytoday.com/us/basics/trauma. Accessed 4 April 2022.

Satchidananda, Swami. The Yoga Sūtra of Patañjali. Buckingham: Integral Yoga, 2012.

Chapter 3

Fromm, Erich. The Art of Loving. New York: HarperCollins, 2006.

McLeod, Saul. "Cognitive Dissonance." Simply Psychology, 5 February 2018. https://www.simplypsychology.org/cognitive-dissonance.html. Accessed 5 April 2022.

Mineo, Liz. "Good Genes Are Nice, but Joy Is Better." Harvard Gazette, 11 April 2017. https://news.harvard.edu/gazette/story/2017/04/over-nearly-80-years-harvard-study-has-been-showing-how-to-live-a-healthy-and-happy-life/. Accessed 4 April 2022.

Ó Tuama, Pádraig, with Krista Tippett.

Bibliography

"This Fantastic Argument of Being Alive." The On Being Project, 2 March 2017. https://onbeing.org/programs/padraig-o-tuama-this-fantastic-argument-of-being-alive/. Accessed 24 May 2022.

Ruhl, Charlotte. "What Is Cognitive Bias?" Simply Psychology, 4 May 2021. https://www.simplypsychology.org/cognitive-bias.html. Accessed 4 April 2022.

van der Kolk, Bessel. *The Body Keeps the Score: Brain, Mind, and Body in the Healing of Trauma*. New York: Penguin, 2015.

Whyte, David. "The Edge You Carry with You." Lecture Series, 2022. https://live.davidwhyte.com/products/march-2022-series-the-edge-you-carry-with-you/categories/2149681828/posts/2155345267. Accessed 1 March 2022.

Chapter 4

Hanson, Rick, with Forrest Hanson. *Resilient: How to Grow an Unshakable Core of Calm, Strength, and Happiness*. New York: Harmony Books, 2020.

Rilke, Rainer Maria. "Widening Circles." Translated by Joanna Macy. The On Being Project, 11 August 2016. https://onbeing.org/poetry/widening-circles/. Accessed 5 April 2022.

WordNet. "Unity." Princeton University. http://wordnetweb.princeton.edu/perl/webwn. Accessed 5 April 2022.

Chapter 5

Encyclopedia.com. "Svadharma." https://www.encyclopedia.com/religion/dictionaries-thesauruses-pictures-and-press-releases/svadharma. Accessed 6 April 2022.

Tippett, Krista. *Becoming Wise: An Inquiry into the Mystery and Art of Living*. New York: Penguin, 2016.

Whitman, Walt. "O Me! O Life!" Poetry Foundation. https://www.poetryfoundation.org/poems/51568/o-me-o-life. Accessed 6 April 2022.

Chapter 6

Lexico. "Dynamic." https://www.lexico.com/en/definition/dynamic. Accessed 1 June 2022.

Satchidananda, Swami. *The Yoga Sūtra of Patañjali*. Buckingham: Integral Yoga Publications, 2012.

Svoboda, Elizabeth. "Why Is It So Hard to Change People's Minds?" *Greater Good Magazine*, 27 June 2017. https://greatergood.berkeley.edu/article/item/why_is_it_so_hard_to_change_peoples_minds. Accessed 9 April 2022.

Wikipedia. "Flip-flop (Politics)." https://en.wikipedia.org/wiki/Flip-flop_(politics). Accessed 9 April 2022.

Chapter 8

Chodron, Pema. *When Things Fall Apart: Heart Advice for Difficult Times*, 20th anniversary ed. Boulder: Shambhala, 2016.

Lexico. "Energy." https://www.lexico.com/definition/energy. Accessed 6 June 2022.

Whyte, David. *River Flow: New & Selected Poems*. Langley: Many Rivers Press, 2012.

Chapter 9

Brihadaranyaka Upanishad, 3rd ed. Translated by Swami Madhavananda. Mayavati: Advaita Ashrama, 1950. https://holybooks.com/brihadaranyaka-upanishad/. Accessed 9 April 2022.

Lexico. "Long." https://www.lexico.com/en/definition/long. Accessed 6 June 2022.

TDB. "Hungry Ghosts...." The Daily Buddha, 26 October 2020. https://www.thedailybuddha.com/hungry-ghosts/. Accessed 6 June 2022.

Tippett, Krista. "Esther Perel: The Erotic Is an Antidote to Death." The On Being Project, 11 July 2019. https://onbeing.org/programs/esther-perel-the-erotic-is-an-antidote-to-death/#transcript. Accessed 6 June 2020.

Whyte, David. *Consolations: The Solace, Nourishment and Underlying Meaning of Everyday Words*. Edinburg: Canongate Books, 2019.

Bibliography

Chapter 11

Jung, C.G. "C.G. Jung: Quotes. Quotable Quote. 'Until You Make the Unconscious Conscious....'" Goodreads. https://www.goodreads.com/quotes/44379-until-you-make-the-unconscious-conscious-it-will-direct-your. Accessed 9 April 2022.

Chapter 12

Greenblatt, Stephen. *The Swerve: How the World Became Modern*. New York: W.W. Norton, 2011.

van der Kolk, Bessel A. *The Body Keeps the Score: Brain, Mind, and Body in the Healing of Trauma*. New York: Penguin, 2015.

Chapter 13

Baldwin, James. *No Name in the Street*. New York: Vintage Books, 2007.

Hanson, Rick. *Hardwiring Happiness: The New Brain Science of Contentment, Calm, and Confidence*. New York: Harmony Books, 2016.

Oliver, Mary. *New and Selected Poems*. Vol. 1. Boston: Beacon Press, 1992.

Psychologies. "Joy vs Happiness: 3 Ways to Build a More Joyful Life," 1 September 2015. https://www.psychologies.co.uk/joy-vs-happiness/. Accessed 9 June 2022.

St. Vincent Millay, Edna. "Still Will I Harvest Beauty Where It Grows." Book Riot, 3 January 2020. https://bookriot.com/poems-about-beauty/. Accessed 9 April 2022.

Welwood, John. *Toward a Psychology of Awakening: Buddhism, Psychotherapy, and the Path of Personal and Spiritual Transformation*. Boston: Shambhala, 2000.

Work That Reconnects Network. "The Work That Reconnects." https://workthatreconnects.org/spiral/. Accessed 9 April 2022.

Chapter 14

Lexico. "Diverse." https://www.lexico.com/en/definition/diverse. Accessed 8 June 2022.

Lexico. "Mature." https://www.lexico.com/en/definition/mature. Accessed 8 June 2022.

Chapter 15

Lexico. "Energy." https://www.lexico.com/en/definition/energy. Accessed 8 June 2022.

Chapter 16

Lin, Kristen. "Life Isn't a Straight Line." The On Being Project, 24 March 2019. https://onbeing.org/blog/life-isnt-a-straight-line-how-to-chart-your-own-river-of-life/. Accessed 3 June 2022.

Index

Index

Index

Sattwa 138, 142
security 14, 18, 30, 32, 43, 47, 62, 78, 124, 136
shadows 32, 45, 55–56, 78, 132
Shakti 139; Chit 122; Icchā 99, 110, 122
Shuddhi 8
silence 32–33, 35, 58, 77–78, 128
Smarana 33, 53, 70
solitude 128
somatic 101
sovereignty 8, 108, 110, 112–113, 132, 135–136, 140
spiritual bypassing 123
spirituality 53, 61
Sraddha 68
stability 45, 67, 101, 140
strength 10, 33, 38, 60, 79, 92, 98–100, 112–113, 122, 139, 152
stress 13–15, 20–23, 26, 60
success 7, 15, 29–30, 36–37, 57, 59–62, 71, 76, 111, 127–128, 132
suffering 15, 22, 75, 78, 91–92, 96, 99–101, 116, 118, 123, 126, 145
support 7, 10–11, 21, 27–29, 41–45, 47, 50, 63–64, 68, 89, 99, 101, 103, 108, 116, 124, 137, 141–142, 144–149, 153
surrender 14–15, 17, 70, 75–77, 86–87, 98, 101–103, 125–126, 136, 140, 152
sustainability 14, 42, 45, 50, 56, 61, 81, 92, 100, 111, 128, 138, 147, 149
Svadayaya 17

Tantra 53
Tapas 17
thrive 40, 46, 61, 71, 91, 95

transformation 99, 101, 103, 107, 135
trauma 15, 21–23, 34, 88, 91–96, 98–99, 101–103
trigger 21, 34, 64–65, 91, 100, 135
trust 9, 17, 35, 38, 41, 43, 46, 96, 107–108, 110–113, 115–116, 123–124, 126–127, 133, 153
truth 5–7, 9–10, 13–14, 24, 27, 46, 48–49, 62, 65, 67–71, 75–78, 82, 87, 98, 101, 107–108, 112, 119, 121, 124, 133, 138, 148

uncertainty 10, 13, 61, 67, 69
unconscious 63, 80, 93, 100
union 5, 16, 18, 33, 40–41

Vairāgya 17, 61, 132
Vāsanā 28, 92–94
Vāta 81, 138, 143
Vichara 109
Vikalpa 104
Vira 36, 122
Viveka 93–94, 99, 109
Viyoga 35
vulnerability 18, 41, 70, 87, 152

warrior 38
weapon 98–107
willingness 14, 25, 33, 45, 70, 102, 108–109, 117, 135, 144
worthiness 30, 45, 76, 88–89, 91, 105, 121, 125
wound 60, 78, 91–97, 98–105, 107

Yama 17–18
Yoga Sūtra of Patañjali 16–17, 25, 64
Yuj 7, 40

175